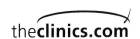

THORACIC SURGERY CLINICS

Management of Stage I Non–Small
Cell Lung Cancer

GUEST EDITOR
Rodney J. Landreneau, MD

CONSULTING EDITOR
Mark K. Ferguson, MD

May 2007 • Volume 17 • Number 2

SAUNDERS

An Imprint of Elsevier, Inc.
PHILADELPHIA   LONDON   TORONTO   MONTREAL   SYDNEY   TOKYO

W.B. SAUNDERS COMPANY
A Division of Elsevier Inc.

1600 John F. Kennedy Boulevard, Suite 1800 • Philadelphia, Pennsylvania 19103-2899

http://www.theclinics.com

THORACIC SURGERY CLINICS
May 2007
Editor: Catherine Bewick

Volume 17, Number 2
ISSN 1547-4127
ISBN-13: 978-1-4160-5141-1
ISBN-10: 1-4160-5141-4

The ideas and opinions expressed in *Thoracic Surgery Clinics* do not necessarily reflect those of the Publisher. The Publisher does not assume any responsibility for any injury and/or damage to persons or property arising out of or related to any use of the material contained in this periodical. The reader is advised to check the appropriate medical literature and the product information currently provided by the manufacturer of each drug to be administered to verify the dosage, the method and duration of administration, or contraindications. It is the responsibility of the treating physician or other health care professional, relying on independent experience and knowledge of the patient, to determine drug dosages and the best treatment for the patient. Mention of any product in this issue should not be construed as endorsement by the contributors, editors, or the Publisher of the product or manufacturers' claims.

Thoracic Surgery Clinics (ISSN 1547-4127) is published quarterly by Elsevier Inc., 360 Park Avenue South, New York, NY 10010-1710. Months of publication are February, May, August, and November. Business and editorial offices: 1600 John F. Kennedy Boulevard, Suite 1800, Philadelphia, PA 19103-2899. Customer service office: 6277 Sea Harbor Drive, Orlando, FL 32887-4800. Periodicals postage paid at New York, NY, and additional mailing offices. Subscription prices are $198.00 per year (US individuals), $292.00 per year (US institutions), $99.00 per year (US students), $253.00 per year (Canadian individuals), $362.00 per year (Canadian institutions), $127.00 per year (Canadian and foreign students), $253.00 per year (foreign individuals), and $362.00 per year (foreign institutions). Foreign air speed delivery is included in all *Clinics'* subscription prices. All prices are subject to change without notice. POSTMASTER: Send address changes to *Thoracic Surgery Clinics*, Elsevier Periodicals Customer Service, 6277 Sea Harbor Drive, Orlando, FL 32887-4800. **Customer Service: 1-800-654-2452 (US). From outside of the US, call 1-407-345-4000**. E-mail: hhspcs@wbsaunders.com.

Reprints. For copies of 100 or more, of articles in this publication, please contact Commercial Rights Department, Elsevier Inc., 360 Park Avenue South, New York, NY 10010-1710. Tel: (212) 633-3813; Fax: (212) 462-1935; e-mail: reprints@elsevier.com.

Thoracic Surgery Clinics is covered in *Index Medicus* and *EMBASE/Excerpta Medica*.

Printed in the United States of America.

CONSULTING EDITOR

MARK K. FERGUSON, MD, Professor of Surgery, Section of Cardiac and Thoracic Surgery, The University of Chicago, Chicago, Illinois

GUEST EDITOR

RODNEY J. LANDRENEAU, MD, Professor of Surgery and Director, Comprehensive Lung Center, Heart, Lung and Esophageal Surgery Institute, UPMC Shadyside, University of Pittsburgh Medical Center, Pittsburgh, Pennsylvania

CONTRIBUTORS

GHULAM ABBAS, MD, Assistant Professor of Surgery, Heart, Lung and Esophageal Institute, University of Pittsburgh Medical Center, Pittsburgh, Pennsylvania

NASSER K. ALTORKI, MD, Chief, Division of Thoracic Surgery; and Professor of Cardiovascular Surgery, Department of Cardiovascular Surgery, Weill Medical College of Cornell University, New York, New York

MATTHEW D. CHAM, MD, Assistant Professor of Radiology, Division of Chest Imaging, Department of Radiology, Weill Medical College of Cornell University, New York, New York

JOE Y. CHANG, MD, PhD, Assistant Professor and Clinical Service Chief of Thoracic Radiation Oncology, Department of Radiation Oncology, The University of Texas MD Anderson Cancer Center, Houston, Texas

BENEDICT DALY, MD, Department of Cardiothoracic Surgery, Boston Medical Center, Boston, Massachusetts

DANIEL T. DeARMOND, MD, Fellow, Section of Thoracic Surgery, Department of Cardiothoracic Surgery, Cedars-Sinai Medical Center, Los Angeles, California

THOMAS A. D'AMATO, MD, PhD, Assistant Professor of Surgery, Section of Thoracic Surgery, Jefferson Medical College of Thomas Jefferson University, Philadelphia, Pennsylvania

TIZIANO DE GIACOMO, MD, Cattedra di Chirurgia Toracica, University of Rome "La Sapienza", Division of Thoracic Surgery, Policlinico Umberto I, Dipartimento Paride Stefanini, Rome, Italy

THOMAS A. DiPETRILLO, MD, Department of Radiation Oncology, Brown Medical School, Rhode Island Hospital, Providence, Rhode Island

ARMIN ERNST, MD, FCCP, Chief, Interventional Pulmonology, Beth Israel Deaconess Medical Center, Boston, Massachusetts

ALI O. FAROOQI, MD, Research Fellow, Division of Chest Imaging, Department of Radiology, Weill Medical College of Cornell University, New York, New York

HIRAN C. FERNANDO, MBBS, FRCS, Department of Cardiothoracic Surgery, Boston Medical Center, Boston, Massachusetts

CLARK B. FULLER, MD, Associate Surgeon, Section of Thoracic Surgery, Department of Cardiothoracic Surgery, Cedars-Sinai Medical Center, Los Angeles, California

SEBASTIEN GILBERT, MD, Assistant Professor of Surgery, Heart, Lung and Esophageal Institute, University of Pittsburgh Medical Center, Pittsburgh, Pennsylvania

SHAWN S. GROTH, MD, Section of General Thoracic and Foregut Surgery, Department of Surgery, University of Minnesota Medical School, Minneapolis, Minnesota

INDERJIT K. HANSRA, MD, MS, Fellow, Pulmonary and Critical Care Medicine, Tufts-New England Medical Center, Boston, Massachusetts

DAVID H. HARPOLE, Jr, MD, Professor of Surgery, Associate Professor of Pathology, Vice-Chairman of Faculty Affairs and Education, and Chief of Cardiothoracic Surgery, Department of Surgery, Duke University Medical Center, Durham Veterans Affairs Medical Center, Durham, North Carolina

CLAUDIA I. HENSCHKE, PhD, MD, Professor of Radiology and Cardiothoracic Surgery, Department of Radiology and Cardiothoracic Surgery, Weill Medical College of Cornell University, New York, New York

ARA KETCHEDJIAN, MD, Department of Cardiothoracic Surgery, Boston Medical Center, Boston, Massachusetts

RODNEY J. LANDRENEAU, MD, Professor of Surgery and Director, Comprehensive Lung Center, Heart, Lung and Esophageal Surgery Institute, UPMC Shadyside, University of Pittsburgh Medical Center, Pittsburgh, Pennsylvania

H. ANNE LEAVER, PhD, Clinical Scientist, Cell Biology Laboratory, Blood Transfusion R&D, Scottish National Blood Transfusion Service, Edinburgh, Scotland, United Kingdom

JAMES A. LUKETICH, MD, Sampson Family Endowed Professor of Surgery and Chief, Heart, Lung and Esophageal Institute, University of Pittsburgh Medical Center, Pittsburgh, Pennsylvania

MICHAEL A. MADDAUS, MD, Section of Thoracic and Foregut Surgery, Department of Surgery, University of Minnesota Medical School, Minneapolis, Minnesota

ALI MAHTABIFARD, MD, Attending Surgeon, Section of Thoracic Surgery, Department of Cardiothoracic Surgery, Cedars-Sinai Medical Center, Los Angeles, California

ROBERT J. McKENNA, Jr, MD, Chief of Thoracic Surgery, Section of Thoracic Surgery, Department of Cardiothoracic Surgery, Cedars-Sinai Medical Center, Los Angeles, California

ARJUN PENNATHUR, MD, Assistant Professor of Surgery, Heart, Lung and Esophageal Institute, University of Pittsburgh Medical Center, Pittsburgh, Pennsylvania

BRIAN L. PETTIFORD, MD, Clinical Assistant Professor of Surgery, Heart, Lung and Esophageal Surgery Institute, Department of Surgery, University of Pittsburgh Medical Center, UPMC Shadyside Medical Center, Pittsburgh, Pennsylvania

ERINO ANGELO RENDINA, MD, University of Rome "La Sapienza", Division of Thoracic Surgery, Ospedale Sant' Andrea, Rome, Italy

JACK A. ROTH, MD, Professor and Chair, Department of Thoracic and Cardiovascular Surgery, The University of Texas MD Anderson Cancer Center, Houston, Texas

RICARDO SANTOS, MD, Clinical Instructor, Heart, Lung and Esophageal Surgery Institute, Department of Surgery, University of Pittsburgh Medical Center, UPMC Shadyside Medical Center, Pittsburgh, Pennsylvania

NORIHISA SHIGEMURA, MD, PhD, Clinical Instructor, Division of Thoracic Surgery, The Heart, Lung, and Esophageal Surgery Institute, University of Pittsburgh Medical Center, Pittsburgh, Pennsylvania

MATTHEW J. SCHUCHERT, MD, Assistant Professor of Surgery, Heart, Lung and Esophageal Surgery Institute, Department of Surgery, University of Pittsburgh Medical Center, UPMC Shadyside Medical Center, Pittsburgh, Pennsylvania

ERIC VALLIÈRES, MD, FRCSC, Surgical Director, Lung Cancer Program, Swedish Cancer Institute, Seattle, Washington

FEDERICO VENUTA, MD, Cattedra di Chirurgia Toracica, University of Rome "La Sapienza", Division of Thoracic Surgery, Policlinico Umberto I, Dipartimento Paride Stefanini, Rome, Italy

WILLIAM S. WALKER, FRCS, Consultant Surgeon, Department of Thoracic Surgery, Royal Infirmary of Edinburgh, Little France, Edinburgh, Scotland, United Kingdom

DAVID F. YANKELEVITZ, MD, Professor of Radiology and Cardiothoracic Surgery, Department of Radiology and Cardiothoracic Surgery, Weill Medical College of Cornell University, New York, New York

ANTHONY P.C. YIM, MD, FRCS, FACS, Professor of Surgery and Chief of Cardiothoracic Surgery, Division of Cardiothoracic Surgery, Department of Surgery, Chinese University of Hong Kong, Prince of Wales Hospital, Shatin, N.T., Hong Kong

JUNJI YOSHIDA, MD, PhD, Division of Thoracic Surgery, Department of Thoracic Oncology, National Cancer Center Hospital East, Kashiwanoha, Kashiwa, Chiba, Japan

CONTENTS

FORTHCOMING ISSUES

RECENT ISSUES

THE CLINICS ARE NOW AVAILABLE ONLINE!

Access your subscription at:
http://www.theclinics.com

THORACIC
SURGERY
CLINICS

Thorac Surg Clin 17 (2007) xiii–xiv

Preface

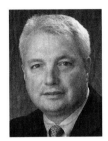

Rodney J. Landreneau, MD
Guest Editor

In this issue of the *Thoracic Surgery Clinics*, we focus on many points of discussion in present and evolving diagnostic and therapeutic paradigms for stage I non–small cell lung cancer.

We begin with discussions of the role of roentgenographic surveillance of patients at increased risk for development of non–small cell lung cancer. Henschke provides us with compelling arguments for the use of "fast," low-dose CT screening for middle-aged persons with significant smoking history and some evidence of chronic obstructive pulmonary disease. Her analysis suggests that such screening is cost-effective in detecting and treating lung cancer at an early, curative stage. She compares the effectiveness of such lung cancer surveillance to that of routine mammography in the detection of early-stage breast cancer.

Advances in percutaneous and transbronchial image-guided diagnostics are reviewed by Yankelevitz and Ernst. The emerging role of molecular biologic staging as a means of detecting a higher risk of recurrence among patients with stage I non–small cell lung cancer by the classic TNM staging system is described by Doctor Harpole.

Roth and Luketich give us intriguing insight into the growing enthusiasm for and the potential emerging role of hyperfractionated radiotherapy and radiofrequency ablation techniques for the small peripheral non–small cell lung cancer. Although most thoracic surgeons continue to disqualify these approaches as reasonable frontline therapeutic approaches to resectable non–small cell lung cancer, other competitive medical disciplines are promoting these interventions as both minimally invasive and effective.

The "can do" individualistic spirit of thoracic surgeons is one of our strongest attributes. Thoracic surgeons may choose to ignore these efforts, similar to the tale of the elephant who sticks his trunk under the circus tent. Rather than despair and cry out, "Who is John Galt?" [1], thoracic surgeons can begin to engage themselves in these percutaneous and radiotherapy techniques. Thoracic surgeons should become fully acquainted with these approaches and establish these modalities as another arrow in their quiver for the treatment of stage I non–small cell lung cancer. Neurosurgeons, vascular surgeons, and urologists have faced similar circumstances over the last two decades, and they have positioned themselves to maintain their leadership position in the management of their particular areas of clinical interest. Just as we profess that our surgical approach to esophageal disease should not be governed by the thin muscular slip known as the "diaphragm," our active, involved approach to curable lung cancer should not be restricted by the presence or absence of a radiation exposure badge.

The utility of sublobar resection for the management of small peripheral non–small cell lung cancers is argued by Pettiford and colleagues. This sublobar resection approach is also described by Yoshida in his appraisal of the management of the peripheral pulmonary "ground glass" opacity. Local recurrence being a primary failure of these sublobar resection approaches has led us to explore the value of adjuvant radiation therapy following sublobar resection. Fernando nicely describes the possible role of intraoperative brachytherapy in reducing this local recurrence event. Maddaus provides us with a contrary point of view in favor of lobectomy for stage I lung cancer, and Rendina gives us insight into the importance of accurate lymph node staging during the course of anatomic lung resection. Rendina also provides further support for the use of mediastinal lymphadenectomy following resection of stage I non–small cell lung cancer.

Thoracoscopic approaches to lobectomy and their merits are described by McKenna and Yim. Walker elaborates on his work in profiling the differences in immunologic suppression between open and thoracoscopic approaches to lobectomy.

The potential role of adjuvant chemotherapy following complete resection of stage I non–small cell cancer is provided by Vallieres. Although medical science, like most other sciences, is "empirical" by nature [2], d'Amato argues that a logical approach to this empiric knowledge be used when suggesting systemic therapy following R0 resection of stage I non–small cell lung cancer.

I invite you to enjoy the contributions of the distinguished and able faculty assembled for this issue. I urge thoracic surgeons to use their individualism, knowledge, energy, and spirit to selfishly strive for improvements in the management paradigms for our patients with curable non–small cell lung cancer.

Rodney J. Landreneau, MD
Comprehensive Lung Center
UPMC Shadyside
Heart, Lung & Esophageal Surgery Institute
University of Pittsburgh Medical Center
5200 Centre Avenue, Suite 715
Pittsburgh, PA 15232, USA

E-mail address: landreneaurj@upmc.edu

References

[1] Rand A. Atlas shrugged. New York: Penguin Group, Inc.; 1957.
[2] Conner CD. A people's history of science: miners, midwives, and "low mechanics." New York: Nation Books; 2005.

ELSEVIER
SAUNDERS

Thorac Surg Clin 17 (2007) 137–142

THORACIC
SURGERY
CLINICS

The Role of CT Screening for Lung Cancer

Claudia I. Henschke, PhD, MD[a],*, David F. Yankelevitz, MD[a],
Nasser K. Altorki, MD[b]

[a]Department of Radiology and Cardiothoracic Surgery, Weill Medical College of Cornell University,
525 East 68th Street, New York, NY 10021, USA
[b]Division of Thoracic Surgery, Department of Cardiothoracic Surgery, Weill Medical College of Cornell University,
525 East 68th Street, Suite M404, New York, NY 10021, USA

Currently, in the United States, approximately 175,000 cases of lung cancer are diagnosed and 163,000 deaths are attributed to this disease annually [1], so that approximately 93% of those diagnosed with lung cancer die of the disease. More than six randomized screening trials have been devoted to early detection of lung cancer [2], but none to date have shown a benefit of either chest radiography or sputum cytology. Japan has provided chest radiography screening for lung cancer for people 40 years and older and has shown a benefit in five case-control studies [2]. These results led the United States Preventive Services Task Force to change its recommendation against screening to being neither for nor against screening. Further, study of the Mayo Lung Project [3] projected up to a 13% increased benefit, and a reanalysis of the Mayo Lung Project results in light of its protocol nonadherence shows as many as 43% of the deaths from lung cancer were prevented [4]. Despite these studies over the past 40 years, the best official recommendation is to be neither for nor against screening.

The introduction of CT screening in 1993 in a scientific study in the United States [5,6] and in practice in Japan [7], however, showed that the proportion diagnosed in stage I can be markedly increased to some 80% to 90% as compared with the 20% to 30% found using chest radiography screening. The three studies performed in the 1990s, all providing both chest radiography and CT, showed that chest radiography missed some 80% of the early stage cancers found on CT [5–9].

Screening for a cancer can be defined as the pursuit of early (latent-stage) diagnosis of the cancer (ie, when the cancer is in its preclinical stage). The purpose of early diagnosis is to provide for early treatment of the cancer, because it is the treatment that serves potentially to prevent the deaths from lung cancer that would have otherwise occurred. Accordingly, the authors partitioned screening research into its components of diagnostic research and intervention research as each requiring different research designs. The key diagnostic question is how frequently are people identified with early stage disease by the screening and the key intervention question is how effective the early treatment is compared with later treatment for early stage screen-diagnosed lung cancer.

This report summarizes the main research questions that have been addressed and their results.

Regimen of screening

The importance of following a well-defined regimen of screening was stated in the initial Early Lung Cancer Action Program (ELCAP) publications on the results of CT screening for lung cancer [5,6]. The requirement for such a regimen was recognized to pool data from many institutions in the subsequent collaboration, the International ELCAP (I-ELCAP), to provide for more rapid evaluation of screening [10]. The protocol specified a common regimen of screening but allowed each institution to specify its criteria for

* Corresponding author.
E-mail address: chensch@med.cornell.edu
(C.I. Henschke).

enrollment [11]. Regular review of the data, updates of the regimen of screening, and pathologic review of the diagnosed cases of lung cancer were performed at the semi-annual International Conferences on Screening for Lung Cancer [12].

The common regimen specified the technical parameters of the initial low-dose spiral CT scan, which were the same for baseline and repeat screenings. The definition of a positive result of the initial CT and the diagnostic work-up leading to a rule-in diagnosis of lung cancer, however, were different for baseline and repeat screenings [11]. Each screening cycle starts with the performance of the initial CT test and ends before the next routinely scheduled rescreening.

For baseline screening, a positive result of the initial low-dose CT is defined as identification of at least one solid or part-solid noncalcified pulmonary nodule 5 mm or more in diameter, or at least one nonsolid noncalcified pulmonary nodule 8 mm or more in diameter, or a solid endobronchial nodule. If none of the noncalcified nodules met the criteria for a positive result or the test was negative, a repeat CT was to be performed 12 months later [13]. Nodule diameter was defined as the average of length and width on the CT image having the largest nodule cross-sectional area. Consistency was defined as solid if the nodule obscured the entire lung parenchyma within it, part-solid if it obscured part of the lung parenchyma within it, and nonsolid if it obscured none of the parenchyma within it [14]. If the result was positive, the work-up depended on the nodule's diameter. For nodules 5 to 14 mm in diameter, the preferred option was to perform another CT at 3 months; if it showed growth of the nodule [15], biopsy, ideally by fine-needle aspiration, was to be performed, whereas if there was no growth the work-up stopped. The other option was to perform a positron emission tomography scan immediately; if the result was positive, biopsy was to be performed, otherwise CT at 3 months was to be done. For nodules 15 mm in diameter or larger (whether solid, part-solid, or nonsolid), immediate biopsy was another option in addition to those already specified for smaller nodules. In instances of suspicion of infection, a 2-week course of antibiotics followed by CT 1 month later was an alternative to any of the previously mentioned options [16]; if no resolution or growth was observed, biopsy was to be performed; otherwise, the work-up stopped. For all cases in whom the work-up was stopped or the biopsy did not lead to a diagnosis of lung cancer, repeat CT 12 months after the initial baseline CT was to be performed.

For annual repeat screenings, a positive result was any newly identified noncalcified nodule, regardless of size; if no new nodule was identified, the CT was to be repeated 12 months later. If one or more new nodules were identified, the work-up depended on the largest nodule's diameter. If all nodules were less than 3 mm in diameter, or if the largest nodule was more than 3 mm but less than 5 mm in diameter, CT 6 or 3 months later, respectively, was to be performed; if no growth was seen in any of the nodules, the work-up stopped. If at least one of the noncalcified nodules was 5 mm or larger in diameter, an immediate 2-week course of broad-spectrum antibiotics was given followed by CT 1 month later. If the nodules showed no resolution or growth, biopsy was to be performed, otherwise the work-up stopped. Positron emission tomography scan was an alternative to immediate biopsy: if the result was positive, biopsy was to follow; if it was indeterminate or negative, CT was to be performed 3 months later; and if it showed growth, biopsy was to follow, otherwise the work-up stopped. For all those in whom the work-up stopped or biopsy did not lead to a diagnosis of lung cancer, repeat CT 12 months after the prior annual repeat CT was to be performed.

The protocol provided recommendations for the diagnostic work-up of a positive result of the initial CT scan; the decision as to how to proceed was left to each participant and the referring physician. The I-ELCAP protocol did not require that its recommendations for the work-up of a nodule be followed. The protocol did, however, require a firmly established final diagnosis of lung cancer and documentation of the work-up in the ELCAP management system [17]. Once the diagnosis of lung cancer was established, the type of intervention, if any, was at the discretion of the patient and physician. Documentation in the management system of the timing and type of intervention, and follow-up in respect to death or manifestations of spread up to 10 years after diagnosis, was required.

Each person diagnosed with lung cancer was classified as a baseline or annual repeat case according to the screening cycle in which the nodule is first identified, regardless of when the diagnosis is actually made. Any case of cancer diagnosed before the next scheduled annual repeat screening is called an "interim-diagnosed" cancer and is attributed to that cycle of screening.

The surgical specimens were examined at each institution according to the I-ELCAP pathology protocol [18,19], which specified specimen preparation and findings to be documented by the pathologist at the hospital where the resection was performed. It also specified the central review process by which a five-member Pathology Review Panel of expert pulmonary pathologists was to reach a consensus diagnosis for each cancer, and to identify lymph node involvement, additional cancers, and pleural, lymphatic, vascular, bronchial, or basement membrane invasion by the cancer.

Adherence to the regimen, however, does affect the performance of the regimen because it determines the frequency of unnecessary biopsy or surgery and the timeliness of the diagnosis, which ultimately determines how early (eg, resectability, stage) the cancer is diagnosed. For adequate performance of any screening regimen, adherence to it by those screened and their referring physicians is important and should be stressed in physician and lay-community education.

Diagnostic performance

In the I-ELCAP experience, a positive result was found in less than 13% of those screened on the initial CT at baseline and less than 6% on the initial CT at annual repeat screening [20,21].

Interim-diagnosed cancers were rare so that the proportion of screen-diagnosed cases was greater than 95% in the baseline cycle and 98% in repeat cycles of screening. The screening regimen turned out to be quite successful as to avoidance of undue invasive procedures, complications, and cost because over 90% of the recommended biopsies according to the regimen of screening resulted in a diagnosis of malignancy. None of the biopsies performed outside of the regimen's recommendation, however, resulted in diagnosis of lung cancer.

The frequency distribution of the cases by relevant prognostic factors, particularly stage of the cancer, is an important performance measure. The authors found that 85% of all lung cancer diagnoses, interim cases included, were of clinical stage I on baseline and annual repeat screening [20,21]. Also, as expected, the median tumor size was larger at baseline than on annual repeat.

The frequency distribution by stage can be used to compare CT with chest radiography when both tests are given to all participants. The marked superiority of CT imaging over chest radiography was demonstrated because over 80% of the stage I lung cancers were missed by chest radiography in ELCAP [5] and the Japanese studies [7–9]. Based on this, chest radiography was no longer performed in the subsequent non-randomized studies.

The I-ELCAP results showed that the smaller the cancer, the more likely it was to be stage I [22]. Although this had always been implicit in the staging criteria, it was questioned in the context of screening and used in part to justify the need for a large randomized controlled trial [23–25]. The I-ELCAP confirmation of the size-stage relationship was also important because it focused the purpose of the diagnostic research on the usefulness of finding latent cancers at small sizes. Most lung cancers without evidence of lymph node metastases are curable, with the curability being higher at smaller sizes [26], and suggest that tumor diameter also serves as a prognostic indicator for curability, perhaps even for micrometastases not detectable by current techniques [22]. Although the authors had previously demonstrated the size-stage relationship using the SEER data [27,28], and a comparison of the screening data with SEER registry data showed that registry data could be used to demonstrate the relationship, it underestimated the real benefit of finding small lung cancers.

The genuineness of these screen-diagnosed lung cancers, particularly the stage I lung cases (ie, meaning that given the opportunity to grow or metastasize because of lack of treatment, while surviving competing causes of death within 10 years), is supported by the panel review by the five pulmonary pathology experts [29]. They confirmed all to be genuine malignancies. Also, for nodules less than 15 mm in diameter, the I-ELCAP regimen of screening calls for documentation of in vivo growth before biopsy [11]. Finally, the untreated stage I cases were uniformly fatal [21].

Intervention research in the context of screening

The aim of the intervention research in the context of screening is to determine the benefit of early treatment in preventing death from lung cancers diagnosed by the screening regimen. Treatment research is profoundly different from diagnosis research because the treatment potentially changes the disease course provided that early treatment is sufficiently effective as compared with later symptom-prompted treatment.

Before the availability of CT screening results, reports based on registries showed 10-year survival rates of 80% in 17 pathologic stage I cases with diameter of 20 mm or less [30] and 93% in 35 pathologic stage I cases with diameter less than 10 mm [31]. The SEER registry, the largest United States cancer registry, showed an 8-year survival rate of 75% in resected pathologic stage I cases less than 15 mm in diameter [32]. Although the lung cancers in the latter three series were not CT screen-detected cases, most were presumably incidentally detected on imaging performed for other reasons in people who were asymptomatic for lung cancer. Using the initial diagnostic research results of ELCAP, the projected cure rate of screen-diagnosed lung cancer was between 60% and 80% [5], which is much higher than what is found in the absence of screening where only some 5%–7%; of people diagnosed with lung cancer are ultimately cured.

For the early diagnosed and early treated patients resulting from screening, the comparator cohort consists of patients who are diagnosed early but treated late, either untreated or only treated after symptoms occur. This comparator cohort provides for learning about the frequency of lung cancer deaths but also importantly the timing of these potentially preventable deaths. This research requires long-term follow-up of early diagnosed patients, both promptly treated or having delayed or no treatment [32,33].

Intervention performance

Actual results from CT screening have now been reported. Sobue and colleagues [34] reported a smaller series of 29 screen-diagnosed cancers that had a 100% 5-year survival rate. I-ELCAP reported the estimated 10-year survival rate of clinical stage I lung cancer detected by CT screening and promptly resected to be 92% and when considering only pathologic stage I to be 94% [21]. It can again be appreciated that the estimates obtained from registry data [26,32], while providing for a lower bound of the benefit of screening, underestimated the benefit.

The proportion of deaths that can be prevented by early diagnosis and early treatment resulting from CT screening is estimated to be 80%, as shown by the overall 10-year Kaplan-Meier survival rate for all diagnosed cases of lung cancer, regardless of stage or treatment [21].

Critics of the authors' study design say that estimates of survival are potentially confounded by lead time, length, and overdiagnosis bias of unknown magnitude, and defy meaningful interpretation [35]. Screening for a cancer, however, is supposed to provide for lead time in diagnosis and treatment. A bias is introduced when treatment effectiveness is assessed by comparing relatively short-term survival rates of a treatment with lead time relative to treatment without lead time; however, the authors did not make such a comparison [21].

The longer the latent stage for a subtype of the cancer, the more prevalent it is in baseline screening. Cancers diagnosed at baseline tend to grow more slowly than the subtype of cancer in general, including when it is diagnosed in the screening's repetitions. Although this fact may call for making a distinction between baseline and repeat screening, it is not a bias. Also, cancers are diagnosed later in their latent course at baseline relative to those diagnosed at repeated screenings, without this being said to introduce timing bias. These facts were reflected in the pathologic findings of the lung cancers diagnosed at baseline and annual screenings [29].

As to overdiagnosis biasing the authors' survival rates, they provided the following countervailing points. Review of the resected specimens by a panel of expert pulmonary pathologists confirmed that all were genuine lung cancer. That review also confirmed that 95% of the resected stage I cancers were invasive, whereas the remaining 5% were classified as adenocarcinomas, bronchioalveolar subtype [21]. This latter subtype by definition does not have invasion of the basement membrane but is considered to be a precursor lesion of invasive adenocarcinoma, mixed subtype. Finally, all those with stage I lung cancer who refused treatment died within 5 years of their lung cancer [21].

Are these results sufficiently effective to justify screening people who are at risk of lung cancer? Compared with mammography screening for breast cancer, the lung cancer detection rates of 1.3% for baseline and 0.3% for annual repeat screening of I-ELCAP participants 40 years of age and older were slightly higher than those of breast cancer of 0.6% to 1% for baseline screening and comparable with those of 0.2% to 0.4% for annual repeat screening of women 40 years of age and older [21]. The cancer detection rate is dependent on the risk profile of the screened such that the higher the risk, the more productive the screening. CT screening of the original ELCAP participants who were former and current smokers 60 years and older [5,6] was more productive in detecting lung cancer because the detection rates were 2.7% for baseline and 0.6% for annual repeat screening. The actual cost of the low-dose CT scan is below $200, and cost of surgery for stage I lung cancer is less than half that of late-stage treatment, so that using the original ELCAP data and the actual hospital costs for the work-up, the authors found CT screening for lung cancer to be highly cost-effective [36,37]. Others have also estimated cost-effectiveness of CT screening for lung cancer for various risk profiles and their estimates are comparable with that for mammography screening [21].

Further considerations

CT screening for lung cancer raises important questions as to the appropriate intervention for small screen-diagnosed lung cancers: (1) is a lobectomy for stage I lung cancer always required or might a more limited resection suffice and, if so, under what conditions; (2) as precursor lesions to some types of lung cancer are identified, what is the appropriate treatment; and (3) what is the appropriate treatment modality for certain types of more slowly growing lung cancer; (4) consideration of possible chemoprevention for precursor lesions; and (5) how should those with multiple small cancers be staged in the absence of lymph node metastases?

Many such staging and treatment questions are being raised at the International Conferences on Screening for Lung Cancer, and for these questions the changes made in the breast cancer staging and treatment provide a useful paradigm.

Summary

A person who is at high-risk for lung cancer and asymptomatic, and who is interested in potentially being screened should be fully apprized of the implications of screening and of the treatment that may result [38]. In light of this, it is reasonable for the individual to choose to be screened by a multidisciplinary medical team with experience in performing such screenings, using a well-defined CT regimen of screening, and having appropriate quality assurance procedures in place.

References

[1] American Cancer Society. Statistics for 2006. Cancer facts and figures. Available at: http://www.cancer.org/docroot/stt/stt_0.asp. Accessed January 16, 2007.

[2] Humphrey LL, Johnson M, Teutsch S. Lung cancer screening with sputum cytologic examination, chest radiography, and computed tomography: an update of the U.S. Preventive Services Task Force. Ann Intern Med 2004;140:738–53. Available at: http://ahrg.gov/clinic/cps3dix.htm. Accessed April 11, 2007.

[3] Flehinger BJ, Kimmel M. The natural history of lung cancer in a periodically screened population. Biometrics 1987;43:127–44.

[4] Miettinen OS. Screening for lung cancer. Radiol Clin North Am 2000;38:479–86.

[5] Henschke CI, McCauley DI, Yankelevitz DF, et al. Early Lung Cancer Action Project: overall design and findings from baseline screening. Lancet 1999;354:99–105.

[6] Henschke CI, Naidich DP, Yankelevitz DF, et al. Early Lung Cancer Action Project: preliminary findings on annual repeat screening. Cancer 2001;92:153–9.

[7] Kaneko M, Eguchi K, Ohmatsu H, et al. Peripheral lung cancer: screening and detection with low-dose spiral CT versus radiography. Radiology 1996;201:798–802.

[8] Sone S, Takahima S, Li F, et al. Mass screening for lung cancer with mobile spiral computed tomography scanner. Lancet 1998;351:1242–5.

[9] Sone S, Li F, Yang Z-G, et al. Results of three-year mass screening programme for lung cancer using mobile low-dose spiral computed tomography scanner. Br J Cancer 2001;84:25–32.

[10] Henschke CI, Yankelevitz DF, Smith JP, et al. Screening for lung cancer: the Early Lung Cancer Action approach. Lung Cancer 2002;35:143–8.

[11] International Early Lung Cancer Action Program protocol. Available at: www.IELCAP.org. Accessed April 11, 2007.

[12] International Conferences on Screening for Lung Cancer. Available at: www.IELCAP.org. Accessed April 11, 2007.

[13] Henschke CI, Yankelevitz DF, Naidich D, et al. CT screening for lung cancer: suspiciousness of nodules at baseline according to size. Radiology 2004;231:164–8.

[14] Henschke CI, Yankelevitz DF, Mirtcheva R, et al. CT screening for lung cancer: frequency and significance of part-solid and nonsolid nodules. AJR Am J Roentgenol 2002;178:1053–7.

[15] Kostis WJ, Yankelevitz DF, Reeves AP, et al. Small pulmonary nodules: reproducibility of three-dimensional volumetric measurement and estimation of time to follow-up CT. Radiology 2004;231:446–52.

[16] Libby DM, Wu N, Lee IJ, et al. CT screening for lung cancer: the value of short-term CT follow-up. Chest 2006;129:1039–42.

[17] Reeves AP, Kostis WJ, Yankelevitz DF, et al. A web-based unsupported reference a system for multi-institutional research studies on lung cancer. Scientific abstract. Radiologic Society of North America; November 2001.

[18] Vazquez M, Flieder D, Travis W, et al. Early Lung Cancer Action Project pathology protocol. Lung Cancer 2003;39:231–2.

[19] Vazquez M, Flieder D, Travis W, et al. Early Lung Cancer Action Project pathology protocol. Available at: www.IELCAP.org; http://ICScreen.med.cornell.edu. Accessed April 11, 2007.

[20] Henschke CI, Yankelevitz DF, Smith JP, et al. CT screening for lung cancer: assessing a regimen's diagnostic performance. Clin Imaging 2004;28:317–21.

[21] International Early Lung Cancer Investigators. Survival of patients with stage I lung cancer detected on CT screening. N Engl J Med 2006;355:1763–71.

[22] I-ELCAP Investigators. CT screening for lung cancer: the relationship of disease stage to tumor size. Arch Intern Med 2006;166:321–5.

[23] Heyneman LE, Herndon JE, Goodman PC, et al. Stage distribution in patients with a small (< or = 3 cm) primary nonsmall cell lung carcinoma: implication for lung carcinoma screening. Cancer 2001;92:3051–5.

[24] Aberle D. National lung screening trial. Available at: http://www1.umn.edu/eoh/NewFiles/nlstinfo.html. Accessed April 11, 2007.

[25] Aberle DR, Black WC, Goldin JG, et al. Contemporary screening for the detection of lung cancer protocol [NLST], 10 May 2002. American College of Radiology Imaging Network (ACRIN sharp6654). Available at: http://www.acrin.org/currentprotocols.html; 2003. Accessed April 11, 2007.

[26] Wisnivesky JP, Yankelevitz DF, Henschke CI. The effect of tumor size on curability of stage I non-small-cell lung cancers. Chest 2004;126:761–5.

[27] Yankelevitz DF, Wisnivesky JP, Henschke CI. Stage of lung cancer in relation to its size. 1. Insights. Chest 2005;127:1132–5.

[28] Wisnivesky JP, Yankelevitz DF, Henschke CI. Stage of lung cancer in relation to its size. 2. Evidence. Chest 2005;127:1136–9.

[29] Carter D, Vazquez M, Flieder DB, et al. Comparison of pathologic findings of baseline and annual repeat cancers diagnosed on CT screening. Lung Cancer 2007 [epub ahead of print].

[30] Buell PE. The importance of tumor size in prognosis for resected bronchogenic carcinoma. J Surg Oncol 1971;3:539–51.

[31] Martini N, Bains MS, Burt ME, et al. Incidence of local recurrence and second primary tumors in resected stage I lung cancer. J Thorac Cardiovasc Surg 1995;109:120–9.

[32] Henschke CI, Yankelevitz DF, Smith JP, et al. The use of spiral CT in lung cancer screening. In: DeVita VT, Hellman S, Rosenberg SA, editors. Progress in oncology 2002. Sudbury (MA): Jones and Barlett; 2002.

[33] Henschke CI, Wisnivesky JP, Yankelevitz DF, et al. Screen-diagnosed small stage I cancers of the lung: genuineness and curability. Lung Cancer 2003;39:327–30.

[34] Sobue T, Moriyama N, Kaneko M, et al. Screening for lung cancer with low-dose helical computed tomography: anti-lung cancer association project. J Clin Oncol 2002;20:911–20.

[35] Henschke CI, Smith JP, Miettinen OS. Response to letters to the editor. N Engl J Med 2007;356:743–7.

[36] Wisnivesky JP, Mushlin A, Sicherman N, et al. Cost-effectiveness of baseline low-dose CT screening for lung cancer: preliminary results. Chest 2003;124:614–21.

[37] Miettinen OS. Screening for lung cancer: can it be cost-effective? Can Med Assoc J 2000;162:1431–6.

[38] Henschke CI, Austin JHM, Bauer T, et al. Minority report: CT screening for lung cancer. J Thorac Imaging 2005;20:324–5.

ELSEVIER
SAUNDERS

Thorac Surg Clin 17 (2007) 143–158

THORACIC
SURGERY
CLINICS

CT-Directed Diagnosis of Peripheral Lung Lesions Suspicious for Cancer

David F. Yankelevitz, MD*, Matthew D. Cham, MD,
Ali O. Farooqi, MD, Claudia I. Henschke, PhD, MD

*Division of Chest Imaging, Department of Radiology, Weill Medical College of Cornell University,
525 East 68th Street, Box 586, New York, NY 10021, USA*

The peripheral pulmonary nodule continues to evolve as a diagnostic challenge. It is being detected with increased frequency, and size at detection continues to decrease. This is caused by a combination of factors, in particular the technologic advances in CT imaging, and their widespread availability. The challenge is to decide on the appropriate work-up. Transthoracic needle biopsy (TNB) is a widely used technique to evaluate pulmonary nodules. This has occurred for a variety of reasons, but primarily relates to improvements in image-guidance techniques. This includes faster scan times with higher resolution, and most recently CT fluoroscopy. Nevertheless, the performance of this procedure is operator dependent and directly relates to the skills of the radiologist to obtain the sample and the skills of a pathologist to interpret the sample provided. To optimize the overall usefulness of this procedure there needs to be careful consideration of the indications and contraindications, followed by choice of equipment to perform the procedure, techniques that improve access to the nodules, postbiopsy techniques to minimize complications, interpretation of the specimen, and follow-up recommendations.

Dr. David F. Yankelevitz is a consultant and shareholder for PneumRx.

* Corresponding author.
E-mail address: dyankele@med.cornell.edu
(D.F. Yankelevitz).

Indications

The indication for performance of TNB in the case of peripheral lung lesions suspicious for cancer is complex, with the need to balance clinical suspicion with the ability to achieve a diagnostic result, and the possibility of performing alternative diagnostic tests. There are two main considerations in regard to suspicion of cancer: the possibility of primary lung cancer and the possibility of metastatic disease. In regard to the former, suspicion is guided by both clinical history and age of the patient. These factors have been well documented as being highly useful in assessing the possibility of a nodule being lung cancer. The recent report of the Fleischner Society [1] includes these two factors in determining whether or not to pursue the diagnosis in a small peripheral nodule. Given a suitable risk profile, however, the work-up for a nodule varies depending on the size of the nodule. The work-up approach that is currently used by the International Early Lung Cancer Action Program Investigators [2] was recently reported. It has a separate regimen for baseline and repeat screening. Critical aspects of the work-up on baseline screening include the recommendation to follow nodules less than 5 mm with repeat scan at 1 year, and for nodules less than 15 mm, to have additional diagnostic work-up before biopsy. On annual repeat scans, all new nodules regardless of size are considered to be growing, and further work-up depends on size or further documentation of continued growth.

Another consideration relates to how well noninvasive work-up can predict that the nodule is malignant so that it may not be necessary to perform a biopsy, but instead the patient could have immediate surgical intervention. Clearly, if the probability is 100% that the nodule is malignant, there is no need for biopsy, and ultimately the use of biopsy relates to making a benign diagnosis. Although there is no set cutoff point for how often the biopsy rate should yield a malignant diagnosis for pulmonary nodules, it has been estimated that from a cost perspective alone the yield should be about 80% [3]. Clearer guidelines have been established for other cancers, and in mammography, if the yield of biopsy is greater than approximately 30% malignant, it is considered that not enough biopsies are being recommended. In the International Early Lung Cancer Action Program [2] screening program, a well-defined algorithm that included TNB yielded a malignancy rate of 93%.

When the suspicion is for metastatic disease, considerations for work-up are based on the type of primary cancer, its propensity to metastasize to the lungs, and the overall appearance of the nodule or multiple nodules. Depending on whether the nodules are first seen along with diagnosis of the original primary tumor, or appear subsequently, the work-up varies. Overall, with the exception of nonmelanotic skin cancer, the work-up for smaller nodules when seen on the initial scan in a patient with known primary cancer is more aggressive than in the context of lung cancer screening. Another important consideration in the work-up for possible metastatic disease depends on the type and effectiveness of available therapy.

Contraindications

Nodule size and location bear on the prospect of obtaining a diagnostic result from TNB. Small size and absence of a direct path in the vertical plane or proximity to major vascular structures all increase the difficulty in performing the procedure. Nevertheless, these should be considered as relative contraindications because virtually any nodule in any location within the lungs is accessible to TNB (Fig. 1). These factors must be weighed by the radiologist in terms of his or her own skill level in deciding whether to perform the procedure. Contraindications to the performance of TNB are for the most part only relative. The only absolute contraindication is an uncooperative patient [4]. In cases where a patient is unable to remain still or follow instructions, the procedure cannot be performed. In such cases, where a diagnosis is considered imperative, performing the procedure while the patient is sedated can be considered. Other relative contraindications include the following:

1. Bleeding diathesis with international normalized ratio >1.3 or platelet count <50,000: When necessary, these can be corrected with transfusion, even on an emergent basis [5].

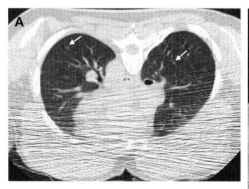
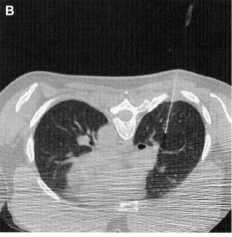

Fig. 1. (*A*) Multiple 2-mm diameter newly identified lung nodules (*arrows*) in a woman with previous history of lung cancer. Prone position, before biopsy. (*B*) Biopsy needle tip located within the small 2-mm nodule. Note that the shaft of the needle is the same diameter as the nodule.

2. Severe pulmonary dysfunction including emphysema or bullous disease: In these cases, careful selection of biopsy path to minimize crossing of severely damaged lung is helpful. Ultimately, these underlying conditions increase the risk of pneumothorax and application of appropriate risk-reduction techniques and knowledge of how to treat the complications is necessary.
3. Contralateral pneumonectomy: The risk in this situation is the development of pneumothorax in the remaining lung. Careful attention to risk reduction and treatment when necessary are the main concerns (Fig. 2) [6].
4. Suspicion of hydatid cyst: Rupture of a hydatid cyst can cause widespread dissemination within the lung and pleural space.
5. Difficulty in positioning: On occasion, patients may have difficulty maintaining a position that allows the easiest access to the nodule. In general, the shortest path to the nodule is chosen for the procedure; however, on occasion the position may be uncomfortable and it may not be possible to maintain for the duration of the procedure. Careful attention to patient comfort before the start of the procedure, and performing the procedure as quickly as possible, help to alleviate this problem. Occasionally, patients must be positioned so that they are more comfortable even though this necessitates an alternative path for the needle to travel that may be longer and more difficult than the original path.
6. Medications with anticoagulant effects: These include warfarin, aspirin, and nonsteroidal anti-inflammatory agents. These should

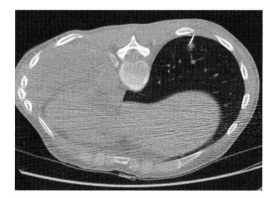

Fig. 2. Patient is status post left pneumonectomy for previous lung cancer. The new nodule in the right lower lobe underwent biopsy without complication. Tip of the needle is seen entering the nodule.

generally be discontinued 5 days before the procedure.

Alternative diagnostic tests

Several diagnostic tests are often considered in the work-up of pulmonary nodules. They range from totally noninvasive, to minimally invasive, to invasive. Under the category of noninvasive, the commonly considered diagnostic alternatives include contrast-enhanced CT scanning and positron emission tomography scanning. There is a large body of literature describing these tests; however, it can be confusing with wide ranges reported for their respective sensitivities and specificities. Some general conclusions about these two approaches can be made. They both have diminished accuracy for subcentimeter nodules. Both are prone to be false-positive with active inflammatory processes, and both tend to yield false-negative results with low-grade cancers. Nevertheless, both of these tests continue to improve as a result of improved technology and are active areas of research and development. Newer high-resolution multidetector CT scanners should impact both of these tests and allow for more accurate diagnosis of smaller nodules. In the case of nodule enhancement, it allows for higher-resolution images of the nodule to be obtained quickly, and this can allow for better understanding of the dynamics of contrast enhancements [7]. In positron emission tomography scanning, newer metabolic agents, such as choline, are now showing promise, and there are many new specialized agents under development. There are also improvements in the scanner technology, notably in regard to hybrid devices with faster multirow scanners. There has also been improvement in respiratory gating capabilities. Under the category of minimally invasive, bronchoscopy is often considered as an alternative to TNB. The published reports of the accuracy of bronchoscopy are nearly uniformly lower, however, than that of TNB. This procedure is generally limited to those cases where there is a positive bronchus sign. This implies that a bronchus is seen leading into the nodule. Even with this favorable sign present, however, the procedure is still less accurate than TNB [3]. Although bronchoscopy is generally used for more central lesions, endobronchial lesions, there have been some major technologic advances that make them more applicable to peripheral ones. This includes the use of CT-guided tracking devices, whereby the location of the tip of the bronchoscope can be mapped to a virtual bronchoscopic image, and the rapidly developing field of ultrathin bronchoscopy that can be guided into more distal branches of the bronchial tree.

Invasive procedures include thoracoscopic biopsy and thoracotomy. These procedures provide for larger amount of tissue compared with TNB. As a diagnostic procedure, however, thoracotomy should generally be avoided. This is a major surgical procedure with associated attendant risks and morbidity [3]. When necessary, thoracoscopy generally suffices to yield enough tissue and can be converted into a thoracotomy if necessary. Nevertheless, early claims of 100% sensitivity and specificity for this procedure have now been found to be incorrect. One of the major challenges from the technical side is the ability to palpate the small nodules or the nonsolid ones. One solution that is gaining in popularity is preoperatively to mark those lesions to allow the surgeon either to see or to feel the lesions more easily. This can be accomplished by injecting dye into the region of the nodule under CT guidance; one commonly used agent is methylene blue. More recently, a technique has been described that uses CT-guided percutaneously injected coils that can be palpated [8]. The noninvasive diagnostic test that is now becoming widely available and is primarily used for assessment of small nodules relies on estimating their growth rates using serial CT scans [9]. This technique leverages the unique ability of CT scanning to make accurate measurements. Once the volume can be accurately measured and the time between scans is known, it is relatively straightforward to estimate doubling times. This technique will continue to improve, and has a role both for the diagnostic work-up and being useful in following nodules where the results of other tests, including TNB, have been inconclusive.

Prebiopsy procedure

Most TNBs can be performed safely on an outpatient basis. Ideally, the images and clinical history are available for review by the radiologist before scheduling the case. The patient should be informed about what to expect before coming for the procedure. This includes a discussion with qualified staff regarding risks and benefits, dietary instructions, medications either to be continued or temporarily discontinued, and to be prepared for the possibility of staying overnight in the event of

complications. It is also helpful to have written or web-based materials available for review that contains information regarding the procedure so that questions or concerns can be considered before the procedure. Laboratory tests are generally required before the procedure to confirm that there are no serious problems related to bleeding. The pathology department should be notified of the biopsy schedule in advance so that they are ready to evaluate the specimen. In addition, many institutions are now requiring documentation of a recent history and physical examination. This can be obtained from the patient's referring physician and must be recent. The radiologist who performs the procedure typically obtains informed consent just before proceeding. The elements of informed consent include a discussion of how the procedure is performed; what to expect both during and following the procedure; the potential risks and benefits, including details about their respective frequency; and potential alternatives.

Patient positioning

The patient position during the procedure is either supine, prone, or decubitus. The choice depends on several factors, including location of the lesion, physical limitations and comfort of the patient, and accessibility based on adjacent or surrounding structures. In general, the position allowing the shortest distance and most direct route is chosen. There are, however, numerous considerations that can alter this choice. Prone position is advantageous for several reasons, the primary one being that there is less chest wall motion. The ribs are attached to vertebral bodies in their posterior aspects and do not move out of the axial plane when the patient breathes. Instead, the ribs rotate in plane. This has been likened to the motion of the handles of a bucket. When the patient is supine, the anterior portion of the ribs moves in and out of the axial plane and this can cause motion of the needle with each breath. The decubitus position has the largest amount of motion because the dependent lung is relatively motionless and most motion occurs in the nondependent lung, which is generally the location of the nodule undergoing biopsy. Another reason to prefer the prone position is that following the procedure the patient is instructed to lie with the biopsy site in the dependent position. This is useful in reducing the risk of developing a pneumothorax (PTX). It is generally much easier for a patient to lie on their back for several hours postprocedure than to lie prone. A final reason for preferring the prone position is that patients do not have to visualize the needle's actual entry. Although many patients simply close their eyes to avoid seeing this, for some it can be quite anxiety provoking.

Additional considerations in terms of positioning relate to ease of access to the nodule. On occasion, there may be structures blocking the path of the needle. This includes bony structures, such as the scapula or ribs, and vascular structures, such as the great vessels. Proper positioning is a major component in planning the procedure and time spent on optimizing this is well worth the effort (Fig. 3) [10]. The scapula can be rotated out of the way by placing the patient's arm at their side and internally rotating the shoulder. This generally moves the scapula laterally. On occasion, it is helpful to place a pillow or folded sheet under the chest so as to allow the shoulder to rotate laterally even further. This technique is also sometimes helpful in spreading the ribs to allow for direct perpendicular access to the nodule without having to advance the needle on an angle to the scanning plane. Regarding the great vessels and clavicle, it is often not possible to rotate these structures out of the biopsy plane. In cases where a nodule is located near these structures, a prone approach is necessary, even though it may necessitate a longer path.

Closely related to the choice of patient position, is choice of entry site. Similar considerations must be given to this as to patient position. Even for a given position there may be choices as to where to insert the needle. In some cases, where structures to be avoided are being considered, such as a fissure, an insertion point that requires a longer route may be preferred (Fig. 4).

Sedation

In general, conscious sedation is unnecessary in the performance of TNB. Most patients are calm enough to allow the procedure to be performed without any additional medication. In addition, it is often desirable to have the patient cooperate with specific breathing instruction during the procedure. On occasion, however, after discussion and evaluation of the patient, it may be worthwhile to administer a sedative. In those cases, it is necessary to conform to all relevant hospital policies.

Breathing instructions

In contrast with x-ray fluoroscopy, real-time evaluation of the nodule while the needle is being

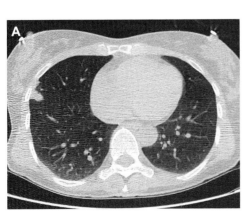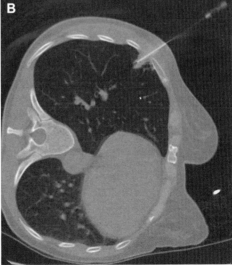

Fig. 3. (*A*) Right middle lobe peripheral nodule. In the supine position, a large amount of breast tissue surrounds the access sites for the needle. (*B*) With the patient in the left side down decubitus position, the breast tissue has moved sufficiently to allow direct access through the chest wall without having to traverse the breast.

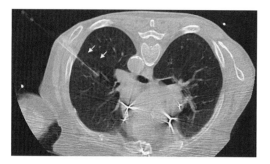

Fig. 4. The needle is inserted obliquely beneath the scapula instead of vertically so as to avoid going through the major fissure. This decreased the chance for pneumothorax. Arrows indicate major fissure.

advanced is not possible with CT guidance. The partial exception to this is CT fluoroscopy. Each adjustment of the needle is performed based on review of the last set of CT images. The needle is adjusted and a new set of images is then obtained. Because there is some degree of respiratory motion, this can be expected to cause some deflection of the needle during the biopsy. In terms of specific breathing instructions, different instructions are given depending on the situation. The main factors that influence this are the proximity of the nodule to the diaphragm and the position of the patient on the biopsy table. The further the nodule is from the diaphragm, the smaller the amount of motion with each breath, and when patients are in the prone position, the smaller the degree of motion of the ribs. Although each situation needs to be independently evaluated, in general, when nodules are located in the upper lobes and the patient can be placed in the prone position the amount of motion in the lungs is quite small and patients are simply requested to breathe gently throughout the procedure. The relationship between the advancing needle and the nodule is sufficiently stable to allow for this approach. When the nodule is located near the diaphragm or when the biopsy is performed with the patient in the supine position, it is often necessary to give specific breathing instructions. Breathing instructions require the patient to suspend their breathing when the needle is being inserted, and also when images are being obtained to check the relationship between needle and nodule. When breathing instructions are given, it is important to rehearse them carefully with the patient so that they fully understand them and have a chance to practice them several times before inserting the needle. Patients are told to

take a small breath, preferably through their mouth, and hold it until instructed to breath. A small breath is recommended because there is less motion of the lung, and when the needle has advanced through the pleura, the larger amount of motion with a large breath can cause increased tension on the pleural surface. It is generally possible to have patients control their breathing so that the nodule is consistently in nearly the identical location for each breath-hold sequence. This allows for the radiologist confidently to advance the needle while not being able directly to assess the location of the nodule. With CT fluoroscopy, the advancing needle can be visualized in relation to the nodule. There are some important differences, however, in comparison with routine fluoroscopy in that only a single axial plane is visualized with CT fluoroscopy and there is a slight, approximately 0.5-second, offset for the images to update. Nevertheless, this technique is quite useful in those cases where there is motion caused by breathing and consistent breath-hold cannot be achieved [11,12].

Preparation for needle insertion

Once the patient has been positioned, a preliminary set of images are obtained to localize the nodule. It is at this point that the relationship with other structures is assessed and an entry point for the needle is chosen. Although patients have already had a set of images reviewed before the procedure and these are the basis for choosing the initial patient position, the relationship of the nodule to adjacent structures can change when their position is changed. This is frequently the case with overlying ribs, and the entry site is only chosen once the patient has been reimaged. The ideal entry point is not always in the image plane that includes the nodule, because there are occasions where planes above or below must be chosen because of a structure blocking a directly perpendicular approach. In general, when a rib blocks direct in-plane access to the nodule, it is better to start above the nodule and angle downward rather than starting below and angling upward. This is because the intercostal vessels run along the undersurface of the rib and should be avoided. To mark the site that has been chosen, a set of images are obtained to identify the plane that includes the nodule. For initial localization a set of markers is then placed on the patient in the chosen entry plane. The entry plane can easily be identified on the patient by use of the laser light that is within the gantry. The markers can be as simple as a set of blood drawing needles taped together and placed on the patient with the axis of the needles perpendicular to the scanning plane. Their purpose is to allow for localization within the scanning plane. A new set of images is now obtained in the scanning plane, with the markers in place. The marker in the optimal location is now chosen. Once the marker is chosen, the laser light on the scanner is then turned on to show the scanning plane on the skin surface and now the combination of the laser light and the chosen marker defines the precise entry site. The skin is marked, generally with a felt tip marker.

With the entry site now marked, the skin is cleansed with antiseptic solution and the surrounding area is covered with a sterile drape. Local anesthesia is now given. It is important to give sufficient anesthesia to make the procedure virtually pain free. This involves numbing by instillation of anesthetic from the skin surface to the parietal pleural surface. There are sensory nerve fibers on the parietal pleural surface, and although it is not necessary to insert the needle directly into it, infusion into adjacent tissue allows for anesthesia to diffuse into the pleura. Documentation of the anesthetic needle adjacent to the parietal pleural surface is useful, and the creation of a small amount of local swelling at the pleural surface caused by the anesthetic agent confirms that sufficient anesthesia has been given. With experience, operators can actually feel when the needle has reached the parietal pleural surface while they are instilling the anesthetic.

Types of biopsy needles

There are numerous types of biopsy needles. They come in various lengths and gauges. Broadly, however, there are two basic types of needle designs that are used: the coaxial design and the single shaft (noncoaxial). Choice between these two is generally a matter of preference. Each type has certain advantages, however, compared with the other. With coaxial technique, multiple samples can be obtained with a single pleural puncture. In this way, if the initial sample is insufficient, additional material can be obtained without the additional punctures of the pleura. The advantage of the single shaft needle is that it is generally thinner gauge, because it does not require an outer cannula, and is more flexible. The

thinner gauge may be helpful in reducing risk of complications, whereas the increased flexibility is found by some operators to be useful in guiding the needle to the correct location. A disadvantage is that when the initial sample is inadequate each additional specimen requires an additional pleural puncture, because the needle needs to be reinserted. This disadvantage is partially offset in those cases where a part of the nodule at some distance from the initial site may need to be sampled, in which case the coaxial approach may not be able to acquire specimen without significant repositioning or reinsertion. Nevertheless, each additional puncture of the pleural surface increases the risk of PTX.

Another distinction between needles is whether they are of the aspiration type or cutting type. Aspiration needles only obtain material suitable for cytologic interpretation, whereas cutting needles obtain material that allows for histologic evaluation. Needles suitable for obtaining histologic material have either a circumferential cutting tip, a side slot that acts as a receptacle, or a spring-loaded cutting edge over a side slot. The spring-loaded needles generally have a throw distance of 1 to 2 cm. In some of the designs, this is adjustable. These needles obtain cores of tissue and are often suitable for histologic evaluation. They are mainly useful for larger nodules and mediastinal lesions where larger amounts of tissue are needed for diagnosis. They can be problematic to use for smaller lesions, because the throw distance may actually be larger than the nodule. In those cases, the tip of the needle has to be outside the nodule before advancing it, and the specimen is obtained without being certain that the tip actually penetrated the nodule.

Needles are also distinguished by the shape of their tips. There are two basic types: symmetric and beveled. Both are sufficiently sharp so as to pass through the skin without an initial incision. The main difference relates to guidance. Symmetric tips tend to travel in a straight line, whereas beveled tips tend to travel in the direction opposite the bevel. Some have found this latter effect useful in guiding or steering the needle (Fig. 5).

Targeting

When the biopsy needle is first inserted, it is placed into the anesthetized soft tissues and its alignment is checked. While there, it can be repositioned multiple times until it is aligned

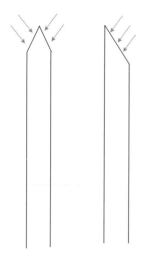

Fig. 5. Different shaped needle tips. On the left is a diamond-shaped tip. Note that the forces that act against it (*arrows*) are symmetric and do not tend to deflect it, whereas on the right, the beveled needle has asymmetric force against the tip (*arrows*) and tends to deflect in the opposite direction of the bevel.

with the nodule, before puncturing the pleura. Nevertheless, it is often quite difficult, if not impossible, to align the needle directly so that it is exactly on course to pierce the nodule. As an example, picture a nodule that is 1 cm in diameter and 10 cm deep to the pleural surface. If the biopsy needle is off target by as little as two degrees, then when it is advanced the full 10 cm, it will miss the target. The smaller the nodules, the higher degree of accuracy required. Although this aspect of aligning the needle with the nodule is challenging by itself, when small degrees of patient motion are added, it becomes apparent that directly targeting the nodule from the soft tissues is generally not possible. A mechanism for changing the course of the needle once it has been inserted, or steering it, is necessary. A technique that is useful for this purpose is often referred to as "bevel steering" [9]. This allows for adjustments without repuncturing the pleural surface. The technique is applied once inspection of the CT images reveals that, on further advancement of the needle along its current course, it will miss the nodule. The steps required are as follows:

1. The needle is partially withdrawn (optional, depending on the distance separating the tip and the nodule)
2. The bevel is turned so that it faces in the direction opposite to the direction that it must move

3. The needle has pressure placed on it to direct it toward the nodule
4. The skin and soft tissues (to the extent possible) are pulled with the operator's free hand to exaggerate the angle of the needle shaft toward the nodule

This approach can cause the needle tip significantly to change its location. The degree of effectiveness is influenced by a number of factors including the depth of the lesion and thickness of the soft tissue. When these are large, there is greater difficulty in repositioning the needle tip. To use this approach successfully, it is often necessary to attempt the steering multiple times. The degree to which the needle is withdrawn and the amount of force placed on it can vary each time. It is an iterative process, in that on the first attempt at steering if there is little movement of the tip, then on the next attempt, the needle can be further pulled back and the torque applied to it can be greater. How much to apply depends on many factors including the depth of the nodule. For peripheral nodules there is little room to pull back without leaving the lung and it may require greater amounts of torque. Once expertise using this technique is mastered, it is possible to make both large and small adjustments to the needle tip location (Fig. 6). When performing biopsies of small lesions, these types of corrections are critically important.

A new type of needle has recently become available that is steerable. It incorporates a set of tendons attached to a joy stick that allow for the needle to flex while it is already inside of the patient. In this way, the trajectory of the needle can be adjusted without having to remove the needle (Fig. 7). It also does not depend on bevel steering, which has a steeper learning curve. Another potential advantage is that the repositioning of the needle tip is primarily transmitted through the distal end of the needle, whereas with the bevel steering approach it is more along the shaft of the needle and may be more traumatic to the pleural surface when repositioning is performed.

Scan parameters

Standard dose imaging for diagnostic purposes is not required for biopsy. Low-dose imaging allows the nodule and the needle to be easily visualized. During the course of the procedure multiple series of images are obtained to monitor the progress of the needle insertion, and the dose to the patient is cumulative with each one. As

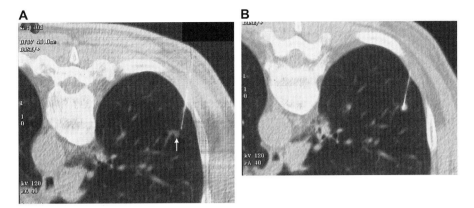

Fig. 6. (*A*) A small peripheral nodule (*arrow*) with needle on a course that would lead to the tip being lateral to it if advanced further. (*B*) Using the technique of "bevel steering," the needle is partially withdrawn, the bevel turned in the opposite direction of the desired movement, torque is applied, and the needle readvanced. The medial deflection is only a few millimeters, but led to a diagnostic result.

a general rule, the lowest dose that allows for evaluation of the needle in relation to the nodule is required. Modern CT scanners can typically have their tube current setting at 40 mA, with some as low as 10 mA.

Slice thickness is chosen in relation to the size of the nodule. A critical part of the procedure is to be able to document the location of the needle within the nodule, and to be certain that a single CT image contains only nodule and is not a combination of lung and nodule, the slice thickness must be at least half the diameter of the nodule. In this way contiguous slices include at least one image that contains no partial volume

effects. A simple rule for choosing slice thickness is as follows:

1. For nodules greater than 3 cm in diameter, a CT slice thickness of 5 mm or larger
2. For nodules between 1 and 3 cm, a slice thickness of 5 mm
3. For nodules between 5 mm and 1 cm, a slice thickness of 2.5 mm
4. For nodules less than 5 mm, a slice thickness of 2.5 mm for guidance and 1 mm for final localization

When performing the procedure, CT images are usually obtained in sets of three to five

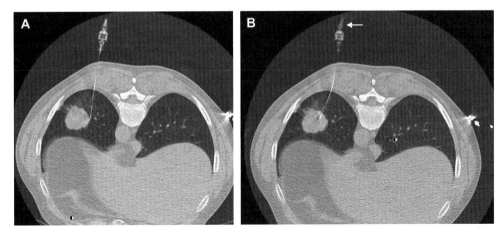

Fig. 7. (*A*) Steerable needle is inserted and the tip of the needle is medial to the nodule in the left lower lobe. (*B*) The joy stick of the needle is flexed (*arrow*) and the needle has now assumed a curved shape, allowing it to be directed toward the center of the nodule.

contiguous images, with the central image chosen to be in the plane where the needle tip is expected to be located, on its being advanced. In this way there are images above and below the needle tip location.

Documentation of needle tip location

Biopsy cannot be successful unless the tip of the needle is actually within the nodule. When specimen is adequate there is no doubt that this has occurred, but when a nonspecific or non-diagnostic result is obtained, there is immediate concern as to whether the needle actually was in the nodule or whether there was a sampling error caused by positioning of the tip. Documentation of the tip actually within the nodule is a critical step in proper performance of TNB, and one that is frequently left out. Documentation of tip location requires following a specific protocol. The first requirement is that images actually be obtained when the needle is advanced and not merely relying on the needle's proximity to the nodule before advancing and taking a sample. It is also necessary to obtain a sequence of images above and below the tip and demonstrate that they include a portion of the nodule. In this way, partial volume effects can be avoided that might give the appearance of the tip being in the nodule when actually it is in adjacent tissue (Fig. 8). Also, when the needle is on an angle and passes through the scanning plane, it may appear that the tip is within the nodule; however, when images above and below are obtained its actual location can easily be recognized. There are three ways to be certain that the needle tip is actually visualized [13]: (1) identification of a distinctive feature of the tip, such as a notch; (2) a long segment of the shaft and hub are seen and there is an intense shadowing artifact that emanates from the distal end (this occurs when the needle is perpendicular to the scanning plane); and (3) images above and below the tip document no additional portion of the needle.

Angled approach

A direct approach, where the entry site is in the same scanning plane as the nodule and the needle can be aligned vertically, is generally preferable but not always possible. Frequently, there are impediments to this type of approach, such as overlying bony structures or large vessels. The problem is even more pronounced with small peripheral nodules because they can have a diameter that is less than the width of a rib and not even a portion of it projects into a scanning plane that does not include the rib. Nodules larger than the width of the rib allow for direct access through an intercostal space, whereas for those smaller, the needle must travel on an angle through the intercostal space adjacent to the nodule. That CT image does not include any part of the nodule. This means that the shaft of the needle is not seen in its entirety from skin surface to the nodule on a single image. The needle passes through successive CT sections until it reaches the nodule. To avoid intercostal vessels, it is generally best to start above the rib and angle downward. In this way the needle only potentially contacts the

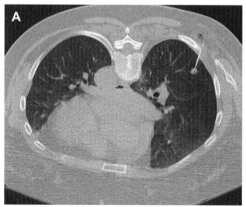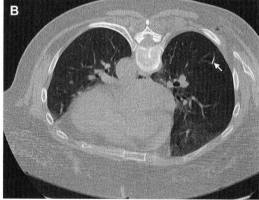

Fig. 8. (*A*) The needle "tip" appears to be entering the nodule on this single image. (*B*) On the image just below, however, the actual tip (*arrow*) is clearly outside of the nodule. This illustrates the importance of obtaining a series of images.

superior surface of the rib. Using simple geometric analysis, the correct angle to position the needle can be estimated by counting the number of contiguous sections that the needle passes through as it advances from the skin entry point until reaching the nodule. By knowing the number of slices and the total length the needle must travel, the proportion of the needle in each successive slice (which is assumed to be equal) can easily be estimated (Fig. 9) [14]. When the nodule is directly beneath the skin entry point, then a single image shows the entire length of the needle along with the nodule. When the nodule is located on a slice next to the skin entry point and when the needle is properly angled and advanced into the nodule, the CT images show half of the needle length in the image containing the entry point, and in the image containing the nodule the remaining half of the needle is visualized. The higher the degree of angulation, the smaller the needle length appears on contiguous slices [14].

An alternative approach is to angle the CT gantry. In this way it may be possible to shift the alignment so that instead of the rib and nodule being in the scanning plane, the intercostal space and the nodule are now in the new scanning plane. In this way the needle can be advanced so that it appears in its entirety in a single plane [15]. This approach avoids the need to focus on geometric considerations related to the scanning plane. The technique is somewhat limited for peripheral nodules that are relatively close to the ribs because the degree of gantry angulation required may be too large.

Diagnostic accuracy

TNB is considered to be highly accurate for the diagnosis of malignancy; however, this is clearly size dependent. For nodules above a threshold size (1–1.5 cm, depending on experience), there is

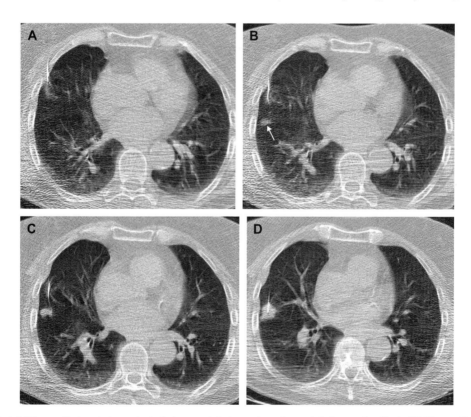

Fig. 9. (*A*) The needle is entering anteriorly in an axial plane where the nodule is not visualized. (*B*) The needle is advancing on an angle upward. Note that the bottom of the nodule is now visible (*arrow*). (*C*) The needle continues to advance upward. Note that the length of the needle seen on each image is approximately the same, and that the nodule is getting larger in size as the needle approaches the center of the nodule. (*D*) The tip of the needle is now located in the center of the nodule.

general agreement about the accuracy of TNB in diagnosing malignancy. It is generally considered to be over 90% sensitive, with less than 1% false-positive rate [16,17]. A recent report showed that for nodules 5 to 7 mm in diameter, sensitivity drops to 50%. Although there have been few reports of accuracy in biopsy of small nodules, there is reason to believe that the failure to diagnose cancer is largely caused by technical factors. There is even reason to believe that biopsy of small lesions may even be more accurate once the technical factors of performing the biopsy are removed. In small nodules there is generally less necrosis and surrounding inflammation and the nodule is primarily composed of actual tumor cells, yielding more diagnostic specimens.

There are three basic categories of results obtained with TNB: (1) diagnosis of malignancy, (2) specific benign diagnosis, and (3) nonspecific benign diagnosis. The diagnosis of specific benign disease is generally more difficult than that of malignancy. In general, this requires a larger amount of tissue for the diagnosis; however, cytologic diagnosis is still possible. Specific benign diagnoses include benign tumors, such as hamartomas; infectious nodules, such as tuberculoma; and noninfectious granulomas, such as rheumatoid nodules. A wide range of results for specific benign diagnoses has been reported ranging from 16% to 68% [5]. These can be explained by three factors: (1) sampling error, (2) amount of specimen obtained, and (3) cytologic expertise. Because benign nodules are generally smaller than malignant ones, it is more likely to miss the nodule and not obtain any representative specimen. Missing the lesion is probably the single most important factor in not obtaining a diagnosis both in benign and malignant nodules [18]. The amount of tissue that can be obtained with cutting needles compared with simple aspiration needles can be substantially different, and in some cases cutting needles provide sufficient additional material to allow for specific benign diagnosis. The skill set necessary for making specific benign diagnosis based on cytology is quite high and not always available; in many situations larger amounts of tissue may be necessary to allow for diagnosis.

The category of nonspecific benign diagnosis is quite controversial. There have been numerous reports that suggest that in the absence of a specific benign diagnosis, malignancy cannot be excluded and a nonspecific benign diagnosis cannot be accepted [19]. This argument implicitly acknowledges that missed lung cancer, even when it is small, is quite serious. Nonspecific diagnoses can be managed with a specific protocol, however, providing that the following conditions are met [20]:

1. That there has been careful documentation of the needle tip within the nodule
2. That when possible, more than a single sample has been obtained from different portions of the nodule
3. That the specimen contains material other than simply blood, such as fibrous tissue or nonspecific inflammatory tissue
4. That a careful plan exists for continued follow-up of the nodule to assess for change

When these conditions are met, the proportion of nodules with nonspecific TNB results that are ultimately found to be malignant is quite low, on the order of 5% to 10%.

Complications

PTX is the most frequent complication related to TNB. This reported rate of occurrence varies greatly, ranging from 15% to 60% [5]. Several reasons account for this wide variation. Earlier reports of PTX rate were based on chest radiograph guidance and in those cases small PTX were not as easily visualized compared with CT. It is possible to see small PTX that may not be visible with chest radiograph and the reported rate may be higher with CT-guided procedures. In addition, patient populations vary and patients who have a larger degree of emphysema have a higher rate of PTX [21]. The choice of needle also affects the rate of PTX. Larger-gauge needles cause more PTX than smaller-gauge needles. Although the relationship between either overall amount of emphysema and gauge of the needle leading to PTX is not exactly known, and there have even been reports suggesting a very limited relationship [22], it is obvious that some relationship must exist and that both of these factors relate to the proportion of patients that develop PTX. Although small PTX generally do not require treatment, if they occur during the course of the procedure they can cause technical problems because of the increased mobility of the lung (Fig. 10). Among PTX that require chest tube insertion, there has also been wide variation in the frequency reported, ranging from 5% to 25% with an average of 7% [5]. Treatment of large PTX is generally required once the PTX reaches

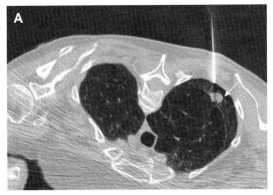
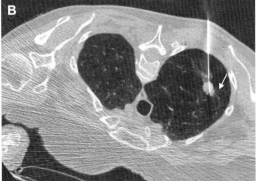
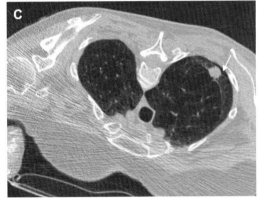

Fig. 10. (*A*) Patient with severe emphysema developed a small PTX (*arrow*) just as the needle touched the pleura. (*B*) As the needle is advanced, the nodule deflects away from it. This can occur with small PTX because it allows the lung to become more mobile and when the lesion is firm, the needle does not easily penetrate it. Note that the nodule has moved several centimeters and its orientation has also changed. The PTX also appears larger (*arrow*). (*C*) Postbiopsy, the nodule returns to its original position. The PTX is now barely visible (*arrow*).

about 30% or the patient is developing symptoms [23]. Treatment of large PTX has been simplified by the development of one-piece self-contained chest tubes that can be inserted by the radiologist. These one-piece chest tubes are easily inserted and allow the patients to remain ambulatory once they are in place. Patients are usually admitted overnight, with most having their tubes safely removed the next day.

Hemorrhage in the lung parenchyma occurs to some extent in nearly all patients undergoing TNB. It results in hemoptysis in only 5% of patients, however, and is generally very limited. Patients should be made aware of the possibility of this occurring before the procedure starts because it can be quite alarming if it occurs unexpectedly. Hemoptysis is usually preceded by a cough. It is generally most severe when large vessels, particularly arteries, are punctured. Although quite rare, particularly with the use of

small-gauge needles, severe hemorrhage is the most frequent cause of death following TNB [24]. Another complication caused by hemorrhage, even in the absence of hemoptysis, is that it can sometimes obscure the target nodule, and makes it difficult to identify them when an additional sample is necessary. This is particularly problematic for nonsolid nodules and because they have open alveolar spaces, they are more prone to bleeding and obscuration (Fig. 11).

Another frequent complication is mild amount of pleuritic pain postprocedure without PTX. In these patients the pain typically lasts for less than 1 hour and is frequently relieved with minor analgesics.

One of the least frequent, but most severe complications is air embolism occurring when air enters the pulmonary venous system. It can lead to systemic air embolism that can cause myocardial infarction, arrhythmia, stroke, and death.

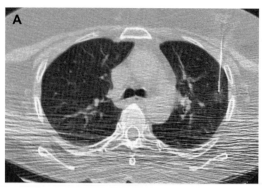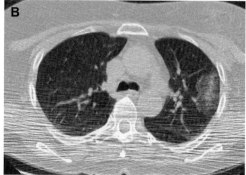

Fig. 11. (*A*) Needle tip is located just above a nonsolid nodule, before specimen being taken. (*B*) After obtaining the specimen, hemorrhage in the region of the nodule has occurred. It also has a nonsolid appearance, and obscures the nodule that it is surrounding. Had a second sample been necessary it would have been extremely difficult to document that the tip of the needle had entered the nodule.

Once air embolism is suspected the patient should be placed in the left lateral decubitus position or in Trendelenburg's position to prevent residual air in the left atrium from entering the systemic circulation. The patient should be placed on 100% oxygen and general symptomatic support should be provided. Patients may then need to be transferred to hyperbaric oxygen units for further treatment [5].

Other infrequent complications include malignant seeding of the biopsy track, which has a reported occurrence rate of 0.012% [25]; vasovagal reactions [26]; and lung torsion following large PTX [27]. Inadvertent puncture of the pericardium can lead to hemopericardium [28].

Postbiopsy routine

A standard set of risk-reduction techniques should be followed postprocedure. There are several techniques that have been used to diminish the likelihood and extent of PTX. The most useful is to turn the patient postprocedure so that the biopsy site is in the dependent position. In this way, the weight of the lung is now pressing down on the puncture site and acts to prevent leakage of air (analogous to compressing a bleeding site). In addition, the alveolar air spaces contract in the dependent portion of the lung making leakage of air more difficult, and there is also less movement of the dependent lung during routine breathing. Patients should remain in this dependent position for approximately 2 hours and are encouraged to breathe normally and remain relatively motionless.

One difficulty with this approach is that for patients who had their biopsy performed in the supine position and now have to lie prone, it is often difficult for patients to remain that way over a long time interval. In such cases, they remain in the prone position as long as they are comfortable and are then allowed to turn onto the side that had the biopsy performed or into the supine position.

Postbiopsy radiographs are ordered to check for the development of PTX 2 to 4 hours postprocedure. If symptoms develop before this, radiographs are obtained immediately. If patients have no PTX at 2 hours and are feeling well, they are discharged after being given explicit instructions regarding development of symptoms and what to do and whom to contact. They are advised to avoid any activity that makes them breathe heavily for at least 24 hours and to avoid strenuous activity for at least 3 days. In patients who do have a PTX noted on the 2-hour radiograph, an additional radiograph can be obtained 1 hour later to assess for stability, provided the patient is asymptomatic. Although there is no absolute cutoff in size of a PTX that mandates treatment, it is generally initiated when the PTX reaches approximately 30% or when the patient is symptomatic.

In patients who develop PTX while still in the biopsy site, aspiration of the PTX can be performed with a small removable temporary catheter, such as a 2-in, 18-gauge intravenous catheter [29]. The catheter is attached to a one-way valve and air is aspirated from the pleural space. Patients are placed on nasal oxygen during this time and it is kept on for at least 1-hour postprocedure. This procedure is nearly always successful in initially removing the PTX and in about half of the patients the PTX either does not recur or recurs to a lesser extent. Among those with enlarging PTX or those who develop it during the recovery period and are becoming symptomatic, chest tube insertion is necessary.

Discharge instructions include an explanation of activity that is permissible over the next several days and a description of symptoms to be aware of that indicates complications. There should also be contact information in the event of an emergency.

Cytology

A critical element in achieving high diagnostic accuracy of TNB is the availability and interaction with the cytologist. The necessity for proper specimen preparation based on the immediate microscopic assessment of procured specimens cannot be overemphasized [30].

Ideally, a multiheaded microscope is used on-site for the evaluation of Diff-Quik stained air-dried smears so that the cytologist and radiologist can view the sample together and decide, based on the evaluation of adequacy, whether an additional biopsy needs to be performed. This decision is not only based on the ability to make a diagnosis but, if benign, whether there is sufficient material for culture and sensitivity studies or, if malignant, for immunochemical studies to assist in determining the primary site of the malignancy.

The initial concern when evaluating an aspirate on-site is the identification of cancer and, if possible, its classification as small cell or non–small cell carcinoma. If mucin is identified in the cytoplasm of the cells or is found extracellularly in the background of the smear, a diagnosis of mucinous adenocarcinoma can be confidently made [31]. When there is an atypical proliferation of bronchioloalveolar cells in a background of inflammatory cells or benign ciliated bronchial cells, an additional sample should be obtained for more alcohol-fixed slides because the subtle nuclear morphology seen in low-grade carcinomas is best seen on Papanicolaou's stain.

Bronchioloalveolar carcinoma is being sampled by aspiration biopsy with greater frequency. Frequently, bronchioloalveolar carcinoma presents as a nonsolid nodule on CT scan. These aspirates yield clusters of bronchioloalveolar cells with small uniform nuclei with finely granular chromatin, pinpoint nucleoli, and intranuclear inclusions and folds. The distinction between atypical adenomatous hyperplasia and bronchioloalveolar carcinoma can be quite subtle and sometimes cannot be made cytologically.

There continue to be improvements in the ability to extract genetic information from small amounts of sample. Currently, amplification techniques allow for microarray analyses to be easily performed on TNB specimens. This may have broad implications for guiding treatment and should allow for an expanded role of this procedure.

Summary

Small peripheral pulmonary nodules continue to be a diagnostic challenge and because of improved technology are also being identified with increased frequency. TNB, performed properly, is a highly accurate procedure and with careful attention to technical factors, nodules of any size in any location may undergo biopsy. A skilled cytologist is an essential part of the team. Continued advances in molecular diagnostics allow for an expanded role of the usefulness of this procedure.

References

[1] MacMahon H, Austin JH, Gamsu G, et al. Fleischner Society. Guidelines for management of small pulmonary nodules detected on CT scans: a statement from the Fleischner Society. Radiology 2005; 237(2):395–400.

[2] International Early Lung Cancer Action Program Investigators. Survival of patients with stage I lung cancer detected on CT screening. N Engl J Med 2006;355(17):1763–71.

[3] Yankelevitz DF, Wisnivesky JP, Henschke CI. Comparison of biopsy techniques in assessment of solitary pulmonary nodules [review]. Semin Ultrasound CT MR 2000;21(2):139–48.

[4] Lalli AF, McCormack LJ, Zelch M, et al. Aspiration biopsies of chest lesions. Radiology 1978;127(1): 35–40.

[5] Klein JS, Zarka MA. Transthoracic needle biopsy. Radiol Clin North Am 2000;38(2):235–66 [review], vii.

[6] Mohammed TL, White CS, Yankelevitz DF. Percutaneous needle biopsy in single lung patients. J Comput Assist Tomogr 2006;30(2):267–9.

[7] Jeong YJ, Lee KS, Jeong SY, et al. Solitary pulmonary nodule: characterization with combined

wash-in and washout features at dynamic multi-detector row CT. Radiology 2005;237(2):675–83.

[8] Powell TI, Jangra D, Clifton JC, et al. Peripheral lung nodules: fluoroscopically guided video-assisted thoracoscopic resection after computed tomography-guided localization using platinum microcoils. Ann Surg 2004;240(3):481–8 [discussion: 488–9].

[9] Yankelevitz DF, Reeves AP, Kostis WJ, et al. Small pulmonary nodules: volumetrically determined growth rates based on CT evaluation. Radiology 2000;217(1):251–6.

[10] Yankelevitz DF, Vazquez M, Henschke CI. Special techniques in transthoracic needle biopsy of pulmonary nodules. Radiol Clin North Am 2000;38(2):267–79.

[11] White CS, Meyer CA, Templeton PA. CT fluoroscopy for thoracic interventional procedures. Radiol Clin North Am 2000;38(2):303–22.

[12] Yankelevitz DF, Davis SD, Chiarella D, et al. Needle-tip repositioning during computed-tomography-guided transthoracic needle aspiration biopsy of small deep pulmonary lesions: minor adjustments make a big difference. J Thorac Imaging 1996;11(4):279–82.

[13] Yankelevitz DF, Henschke CI. Needle-tip localization for CT-guided biopsies. J Thorac Imaging 1993;8(3):241–3.

[14] Yankelevitz DF, Henschke CI, Davis SD. Percutaneous CT biopsy of chest lesions: an in vitro analysis of the effect of partial volume averaging on needle positioning. AJR Am J Roentgenol 1993;161(2):273–8.

[15] Stern EJ, Webb WR, Gamsu G. CT gantry tilt: utility in transthoracic fine-needle aspiration biopsy. Work in progress. Radiology 1993;187(3):873–4.

[16] Taft PD, Szyfelbein WM, Greene R. A study of variability in cytologic diagnoses based on pulmonary aspiration specimens. Am J Clin Pathol 1980;73(1):36–40.

[17] Wallace MJ, Krishnamurthy S, Broemeling LD, et al. CT-guided percutaneous fine-needle aspiration biopsy of small (< or = 1-cm) pulmonary lesions. Radiology 2002;225(3):823–8.

[18] Westcott JL. Needle biopsy of chest lesions. In: Taveras JM, Ferrucci JT, editors. Radiology, vol. 1. Philadelphia: JB Lippincott; 1995; Chapter 45.

[19] Liptay MJ. Solitary pulmonary nodule: treatment options. Chest 1999;116(6 Suppl):517S–8S.

[20] Yankelevitz DF, Henschke CI, Koizumi JH, et al. CT-guided transthoracic needle biopsy of small solitary pulmonary nodules. Clin Imaging 1997;21(2):107–10.

[21] Miller KS, Fish GB, Stanley JH, et al. Prediction of pneumothorax rate in percutaneous needle aspiration of the lung. Chest 1988;93(4):742–5.

[22] Cox JE, Chiles C, McManus CM, et al. Transthoracic needle aspiration biopsy: variables that affect risk of pneumothorax. Radiology 1999;212(1):165–8.

[23] Moore EH. Needle-aspiration lung biopsy: a comprehensive approach to complication reduction. J Thorac Imaging 1997;12(4):259–71.

[24] Protopapaz Z, White CS, Miller BH, et al. Transthoracic needle biopsy: results of a nationwide survey [abstract]. Radiology 1996;201(P):270–1.

[25] Ayar D, Golla B, Lee JY, et al. Needle-track metastasis after transthoracic needle biopsy. J Thorac Imaging 1998;13(1):2–6.

[26] Moore EH. Technical aspects of needle aspiration lung biopsy: a personal perspective. Radiology 1998;208(2):303–18.

[27] Fogarty JP, Dudek G. An unusual case of lung torsion [review]. Chest 1995;108(2):575–8.

[28] Man A, Schwarz Y, Greif J. Case report: cardiac tamponade following fine needle aspiration (FNA) of a mediastinal mass. Clin Radiol 1998;53(2):151–2.

[29] Yankelevitz DF, Davis SD, Henschke CI. Aspiration of a large pneumothorax resulting from transthoracic needle biopsy. Radiology 1996;200(3):695–7.

[30] Vazquez MF, Yankelevitz DF. The radiologic appearance of solitary pulmonary nodules and their cytologic-histologic correlation [review]. Semin Ultrasound CT MR 2000;21(2):149–62.

[31] Roger V, Nasiell M, Linden M, et al. Cytologic differential diagnosis of bronchiolo-alveolar carcinoma and bronchogenic carcinoma. Acta Cytol 1976;20:303–7.

Thorac Surg Clin 17 (2007) 159–165

Bronchoscopic-Directed Diagnosis of Peripheral Lung Lesions Suspicious for Cancer

Inderjit K. Hansra, MD, MS[a], Armin Ernst, MD, FCCP[b],*

[a]*Pulmonary and Critical Care Medicine, Tufts-New England Medical Center,
750 Washington Street, Box 369, Boston, MA 02111, USA*
[b]*Interventional Pulmonology, Beth Israel Deaconess Medical Center, 330 Brookline Avenue,
Boston, MA 02115, USA*

Bronchoscopy has been used for over 30 years in the evaluation of solitary pulmonary nodules and peripheral lung masses [1,2]. Transbronchial biopsy, an approach that uses a biopsy forceps to obtain lung tissue beyond the field of vision, has been the approach most used in attempting this diagnosis. The yield of transbronchial biopsies is substantially better if the lesion is central and large in size [3,4]. Diagnosing a malignant process by bronchoscopy in a small, peripheral nodule has proved to be very difficult. For nodules less than 1.5 cm in diameter, the sensitivity of bronchoscopy for detecting a malignant process may be as low as 10%. If the CT scan reveals a bronchus leading directly to the lesion, bronchoscopy has about 70% sensitivity [5]. Several factors may increase the sensitivity in peripheral lesion, including the use of fluoroscopy with transbronchial biopsies (TBBX) and presence of rapid visualization by an on-site cytologist. Unfortunately, small nodules may not be visualized by fluoroscopy, and a negative result obtained by transbronchial biopsies does not necessarily rule out malignancy.

The American College of Chest Physicians Lung Cancer Guidelines [6] do not recommend bronchoscopy in patients with solitary pulmonary nodules, qualifying the level of evidence as good; benefit, none; and grade of recommendation, D. Transthoracic needle aspiration was also not recommended except in patients who decline surgical intervention or who are not operable candidates. Recent technical advances have become available that may have the potential of increasing the diagnostic accuracy of bronchoscopy, however, and may lead to less invasive methods of diagnosing peripheral intrapulmonary lesions. Based on these new innovations, the role of bronchoscopy in diagnosing peripheral lesions needs to be re-examined.

Advantages of a bronchoscopic approach

Bronchoscopy is a minimally invasive approach that does not subject the patient to potential complications of general anesthesia. The mortality for bronchoscopy is 1 in 4000, with a complication rate for pneumothorax after bronchoscopy with transbronchial biopsy of approximately 2%. Most bronchoscopists currently use moderate sedation during the procedure, which when used by trained personnel is exceedingly safe. The alternative to bronchoscopy is a CT-guided fine-needle aspiration or a primary surgical procedure, such as video-assisted thoracic surgery or thoracotomy. CT-guided fine-needle aspiration has a much higher complication rate of pneumothorax than bronchoscopy, with an incidence of up to 30% [3]. Moreover, most patients diagnosed with a peripheral lung lesion have some degree of emphysematous change or poor pulmonary function, which may explain the increased risk for pneumothorax by percutaneous techniques. Thoracic surgery has the obvious disadvantages of the patient having to undergo general anesthesia, the presence of a surgical

---

* Corresponding author.
 E-mail address: aernst@bidmc.harvard.edu (A. Ernst).

wound, and the need to tolerate single lung ventilation during the procedure. Mortality for this
procedure can be as high as 2% [7,8]. To save patients from undergoing more surgical procedures,
especially if no benefit is associated with the surgical removal of the tissue in question, new imaging
and guidance technology have recently been developed for bronchoscopists. Once mastered,
these techniques may help bronchoscopists in
evaluating peripheral lesions with better diagnostic accuracy.

CT-guided bronchoscopy

CT-guided bronchoscopy is a natural out-
growth of conventional fluoroscopy guidance for
bronchoscopic procedures. Newer CT scanning
equipment is frequently enabled to perform CT-
fluoroscopic imaging, which allows for the exact
placement and steering of percutaneous biopsies
by radiologists. The image provides a CT-slice
view rather than the anteroposterior imaging seen
on conventional fluoroscopy. CT fluoroscopic
guidance has been described as a successful technique for guidance of bronchoscopic transbronchial needle biopsy [9]. It can also be used for
transbronchial biopsies, but there is little published in the literature for this approach.

When using this technology, the patient is
placed into an appropriate scanner and a pilot
CT is obtained through the areas of interest. For
TBBX, a flexible forceps is introduced through
a bronchoscope channel and is advanced through
the bronchial branches to the peripheral lesion in
the axial plane with CT guidance. The forceps is
subsequently opened and CT scan confirms contact with the lesion before biopsies are taken
(quick-check) (Figs. 1–3).

The disadvantages of this technique are the
logistics involved and the radiation exposure to
the patient and the staff. It may be difficult to
book valuable CT time for the bronchoscopy and
the endoscopic equipment has to be transferred
into the room. In the authors' hands, the average
time of CT room use for a CT-guided bronchoscopy is 45 minutes.

The radiation exposure is somewhat difficult to
quantify, because it depends on many variables. It
probably depends most directly on the total
fluoroscopy time used. When used at the authors'
institution, the average fluoroscopy time is
20 seconds per case using a quick-check technique. Even though easy to learn and intuitive

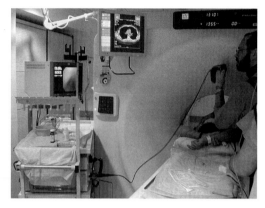

Fig. 1. Basic room setup for CT fluoroscopy–guided
transbronchial biopsy. Endoscopic screens and fluoroscopy screens are next to each other, and the radiologic image is obtained by the use of a foot pedal during the
procedure. (*From* Schwarz Y, Greif J, Becker HD, et al.
Real-time electromagnetic navigation bronchoscopy to peripheral lesions using overlaid CT images: the first human
study. Chest 2006;129:989; with permission. Copyright
© 2006 by the American College of Chest Physicians.)

with a good success rate, this technique may be
logistically too cumbersome for use at most
institutions and radiation exposure issues are
important to address.

**Endobronchial ultrasound–guided transbronchial
lung biopsy**

Endoscopic ultrasound was originally developed to provide imaging guidance to diagnose

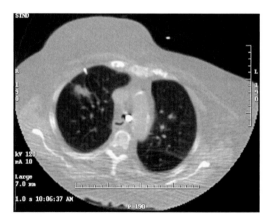

Fig. 2. Image of a peripheral lesion and the tip of a biopsy forceps. The tip is at the pleural surface and a biopsy would not obtain a diagnosis and probably result
in a pneumothorax. Note that conventional fluoroscopic
anteroposterior imaging would most likely have shown
the forceps to be within the lesion.

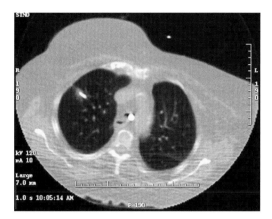

Fig. 3. Image of the same peripheral lesion as in Fig. 2. The forceps is clearly visible with in the lesion.

gastrointestinal lesions. The difference in resistance of various tissues to the ultrasonic waves (impedance) allows for the visualization of soft tissues. In the past decade, the probes have been miniaturized to allow passage through the bronchoscope [10,11]. In the central airways, a radial 20-MHz probe with a balloon at the tip provides a 360-degree image of the airway wall, parabronchial, and paratracheal structures (Fig. 4). Under favorable conditions, a depth of 4 cm can be penetrated clearly visualizing parabronchial and mediastinal structures. These probes can be advanced into regular flexible bronchoscopes that have a biopsy channel at least 2.6 mm in diameter.

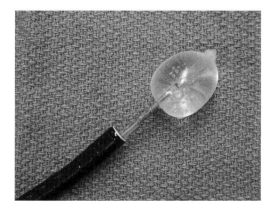

Fig. 4. Image of a radial ultrasound probe advanced through the working channel of a bronchoscope. A balloon surrounding the transducer is filled with water or saline and can be inflated. This serves the purpose of achieving "coupling" to the tissues of interest within the airways. This balloon does not require inflation when used in the lung periphery, because good image is obtained when a solid structure is entered or the probe abuts it laterally.

Although this technique can be used for the successful guidance of transbronchial needle aspiration of mediastinal nodes [12,13], it is quite cumbersome and involves the visualization of the node, removal of the probe, and then puncture of the observed abnormal lymph node with the help of dedicated needles. A newer bronchoscope made by Olympus (XBF-UC40P, Olympus, Melville, New York) is dedicated to the use of transbronchial needle aspiration only (Fig. 5). The tip of the scope has an integrated digital ultrasound array and through a biopsy channel of 2 mm, needles can be advanced and the lymph node puncture observed and controlled in a real-time manner. Endobronchial ultrasound (EBUS) allows for guidance without radiation exposure to the patient or staff. EBUS has long been used with transbronchial needle aspiration in the diagnosis of mediastinal lymph nodes and preoperative staging. This procedure has been especially helpful in improving the results of N-staging of lung cancer.

Recently, EBUS by the radial probe has been used in locating and diagnosing peripheral intrapulmonary lesions [14,15]. The probe is advanced though the working channel similar to other tools, such as forceps, into the periphery. This application is not intuitive, because air acts as an insulator for ultrasound waves and application within air-filled spaces, such as the lung, does not seem feasible. When advanced into healthy, normal lungs, the EBUS image obtained by radial probes has been likened to a "snowstorm" (Fig. 6). The

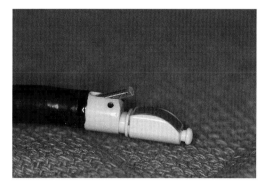

Fig. 5. Distal tip of a dedicated transbronchial needle aspiration endobronchial ultrasound (EBUS) bronchoscope (Olympus Corporation, Melville, New York). The digital array is visible at the distal end and a sheathed needle is exiting at a 30-degree angle from the bronchoscope. The needle entry can be observed under real-time conditions.

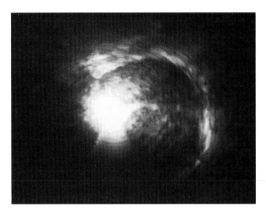

Fig. 6. Typical EBUS image of air-filled lung. No specific structures can be visualized. The image has been likened to a "snowstorm."

principle used is that soft tissue images obtained in the lungs by the ultrasound probe must come from solid structures, such as nodules and masses (Fig. 7).

In an early prospective study comparing EBUS-guided TBBX, with TBBX with fluoroscopy to diagnose peripheral lung lesions, EBUS was found to be equivalent to fluoroscopy without the radiation exposure associated with fluoroscopy [15]. In this particular study, 50 consecutive patients were examined and the mean diameter of the lesions was 3.31 ± 0.92 cm. All patients without a definitive diagnosis underwent a surgical

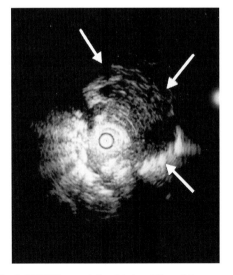

Fig. 7. EBUS in a peripheral lesion. The solid structures of the lesion are clearly identifiable (arrows).

biopsy. Not surprisingly, yield continued to depend significantly on the size of the lesions and for all comers was 80%. A trend emerged for lesions less than 3 cm in size to be found more often when EBUS was used, but this trend was not significant.

Based on the described study, a follow-up study was performed specifically to examine if the use of EBUS can be helpful in lesions that cannot be visualized by fluoroscopy [16]. This is not an uncommon circumstance and generally leads to the cancellation of a planned procedure. In this study, 35 patients were enrolled who at the onset of a planned bronchoscopy with TBBX were found to have nodules that were invisible by fluoroscopy. EBUS was performed with the help of the radial probe as before. A guide sheath was used that was left in place if localization by EBUS was successful and then could be used to advance the forceps into the same area. Lesions were localized in 89% of patients, and diagnostic biopsy tissue was obtained in 70% of patients. These are patients whose procedure may have otherwise been cancelled and, importantly, the biopsy results prevented the need for surgery in 17% of patients. This report is one of the first indicating that newer technologies can be superior to use of conventional fluoroscopy and that a significant number of patients do not require more expensive and invasive surgical biopsy procedures.

Another prospective study by another group compared the accuracy of EBUS-TBBX versus TBBX alone in peripheral lung lesions less than 3 cm in diameter. In peripheral lesions less than 3 cm in size, EBUS-TBBX was much more sensitive and accurate than TBBX alone, once again confirming that EBUS guidance is very useful in diagnosing peripheral lung lesions that previously may have eluded bronchoscopists [14]. Pulmonologists have become more and more innovative in their use of EBUS to diagnose peripheral lung lesions. In the coming years, the more experience that is obtained using this technique, the more accurate and helpful this system will be in aiding in the diagnosis of peripheral lung lesions.

Electromagnetic navigation during flexible bronchoscopy

Electromagnetic navigation is an image-guided localization device that assists in placing endobronchial tools in the desired areas of the lung. This electromagnetic navigation system or superDimension/Bronchus system (SDBS) (super-Dimension, Herzliya, Israel) uses low-frequency electromagnetic waves emitted from a board placed under the cephalad end of the bronchoscopy table (Fig. 8). The patient's chest is within the electromagnetic field and tools equipped with special sensors used by the bronchoscope can be tracked in that field. Because electromagnetic waves are used, the system cannot be used on patients with such devices as pacemakers or automatic implantable cardioverter-defibrillators.

A 1-mm diameter, 8-mm long sensor probe is attached to the tip of a flexible metal cable, also called the locatable guide. Movement of the tool in the X, Y, and Z planes and the orientation (pitch, roll, and yaw) is tracked through the electromagnetic field and captured by the system. The information about location, orientation, and movement is then superimposed on a virtual endoscopic environment based on a previously acquired CT scan and is displayed on a monitor in real-time. To allow for active steering to the intended target, the locatable guide has a built-in bending mechanism that allows for the tip to be aimed in multiple different directions while advancing the tools (Fig. 9).

Navigation of the instrument requires several steps. First, the procedure needs to be carefully planned. This occurs in the virtual environment created from the CT dataset. The bronchoscopy is basically simulated before the actual procedure and the tract is planned. The quality of the virtual

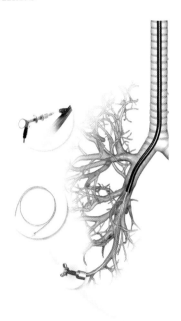

Fig. 9. Composite image showing the steering handle of the locatable guide, the locatable guide by itself, and a forceps passed through the guidance sheath after navigation to the target. (*From* Schwarz Y, Greif J, Becker HD, et al. Real-time electromagnetic navigation bronchoscopy to peripheral lesions using overlaid CT images: the first human study. Chest 2006;129:990; with permission. Copyright © 2006 by the American College of Chest Physicians.)

environment is dependent on the quality of the CT scan and care must be taken to plan the procedure in good detail. The next step is alignment of the virtual plan with the patient's actual anatomy during the bronchoscopy. This is achieved by having assigned landmarks during the virtual planning, which are easily recognized during the endoscopy (usually carinas) and also marked, or "registered," in the same location. The computer software then automatically aligns both environments.

The navigation for the most part is based on the environment visible on the computer screen that allows the bronchoscopist to navigate in three-dimensional reconstructed CT images of the subject's anatomy in coronal, sagittal, and axial views (Fig. 10) [17].

The fully retractable probe is incorporated into a 130-cm long, 1.9-mm diameter flexible catheter or sheath. Once the area of interest in reached, the locatable guide with the sensor is removed and the guide sheath stays in place, allowing for multiple

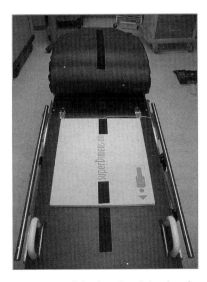

Fig. 8. Placement of the board emitting low-frequency electromagnetic waves on the examination table.

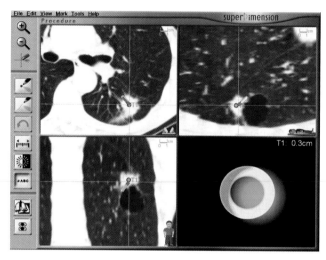

Fig. 10. Typical image of the navigation screen. The location of the tip is visible in three conventional views, and a "forward view" as seen in the lower right hand corner. The "bulls- eye" indicates that the target is in straight view and the distance to the target is indicated as 0.3 cm.

tools and endoscopic accessories to be passed. Among those accessories, the authors routinely use a radial EBUS. This allows for final confirmation that the goal has been reached. It is important to remember that the electromagnetic guidance is based on CT images obtained before the examination, and that navigation is not strictly real-time. Endobronchial ultrasound or fluoroscopic confirmation of appropriate location is at this stage still a necessary feature of the system.

Currently, when attempting to diagnose peripheral lung lesions with the flexible bronchoscope, forceps are guided to the general direction of the lesion, but there is no guarantee that the forceps actually reach the lesion. The ability to guide the locatable guide in three dimensions allows for the localization of these nodules or infiltrates and a steerable probe that allows for active manipulation within the airways [18]. This should improve the diagnostic accuracy.

The first human study was a prospective controlled study published in 2006. Thirteen of 15 subjects enrolled underwent the SDBS navigation procedure for peripheral lung lesions ranging in size from 1.5 to 5 cm, which were beyond the optical reach of the bronchoscope. Four of the lesions were in the left upper lobe, three at the right upper lobe, five at the right lower lobe, and one at the right middle lobe. In 9 (69%) of the 13 subjects, a definitive diagnosis was established. No device-related adverse events were reported during or up to 48 hours after the study [19].

After several studies advocating the usage of SDBS in animals, this study was the first one of its kind in human subjects.

More recently, a larger prospective study involving 60 patients was performed to determine the ability of this technology to diagnose peripheral lung lesions and mediastinal lymph nodes [20]. The mean size of the pulmonary nodules was 22.8 ± 12.6 mm, although 57% of lesions were less than 20 mm. The diagnostic yield was 74% and not significantly affected by lesion size. The diagnosis was obtained in 80.3% of all procedures (including lymph node sampling). Pneumothorax occurred in two (3.5%) patients who had transbronchial biopsies of lesions that were in upper lobe locations. Because of its high diagnostic sensitivity, this procedure once properly learned may have the potential to allow patients to undergo less invasive testing for peripheral lesions in the future. As a caveat, it is necessary to point out that most reports still use additional imaging guidance, such as fluoroscopy and EBUS, and the system has not been tested head to head with those technologies to show and prove the added benefit.

Summary

Bronchoscopic techniques have come a long way in diagnosing peripheral lung lesions suspicious for cancer. Following in the footsteps of gastrointestinal endoscopy, bronchoscopy has become more useful in diagnosing lesions previously thought to be unreachable. The procedure has required miniaturization of the tools used for diagnosis and, as these tools become more sophisticated, bronchoscopists are better able to reach these lesions noninvasively. EBUS has allowed biopsy and penetration with direct visualization of the needle as it enters the lesion. Although EBUS has been used extensively in diagnosing and staging mediastinal lymph nodes, the authors believe this technique has great promise in diagnosing peripheral lung lesions not visualized by fluoroscopy. Electromagnetic navigation adds an entire new dimension to the field of bronchoscopy. The ability to navigate through the bronchial tree in three dimensions and the locatable guide, which is steerable, allow the bronchoscopist to reach peripheral lesions with great success. This technology has great promise in not only diagnosing peripheral lung lesions with greater accuracy, but also may provide a means for therapeutic interventions through this minimally invasive technique. Patients with peripheral lung lesions may now be diagnosed more reliable through endoscopic techniques, avoiding unnecessary surgery in many cases.

References

[1] Torrington KG, Kern JD. The utility of fiberoptic bronchoscopy in the evaluation of the solitary pulmonary nodule. Chest 1993;104(4):1021–4.

[2] Wallace JM, Deutsch AL. Flexible fiberoptic bronchoscopy and percutaneous needle lung aspiration for evaluating the solitary pulmonary nodule. Chest 1982;81(6):665–71.

[3] Tan BB, Flaherty KR, Kazerooni EA, et al. The solitary pulmonary nodule. Chest 2003;123(1 Suppl): 89S–96S.

[4] Baaklini WA, Reinoso MA, Gorin AB, et al. Diagnostic yield of fiberoptic bronchoscopy in evaluating solitary pulmonary nodules. Chest 2000;117(4):1049–54.

[5] Ost D, Fein AM, Feinsilver SH. Clinical practice: the solitary pulmonary nodule. N Engl J Med 2003;348(25):2535–42.

[6] Diagnosis and management of lung cancer: ACCP evidence-based guidelines. American College of Chest Physicians. Chest 2003;123(1 Suppl): D-G, 1S–337S.

[7] Walker WS, Codispoti M, Soon SY, et al. Long-term outcomes following VATS lobectomy for non-small cell bronchogenic carcinoma. Eur J Cardiothorac Surg 2003;23(3):397–402.

[8] Allen MS, Pairolero PC. Inadequacy, mortality, and thoracoscopy. Ann Thorac Surg 1995;59(1):6.

[9] Garpestad E, Goldberg NS, Herth F, et al. CT fluoroscopy guidance for transbronchial needle aspiration: an experience in 35 patients. Chest 2001;119:329–32.

[10] Herth FJ, Ernst A. Innovative bronchoscopic diagnostic techniques: endobronchial ultrasound and electromagnetic navigation. Curr Opin Pulm Med 2005;11(4):278–81.

[11] Feller-Kopman D, Lunn W, Ernst A. Autofluorescence bronchoscopy and endobronchial ultrasound: a practical review. Ann Thorac Surg 2005;80(6): 2395–401.

[12] Herth FJ, Eberhardt R, Vilmann P, et al. Real-time, endobronchial ultrasound-guided, transbronchial needle aspiration: a new method for sampling mediastinal lymph nodes. Thorax 2006;61(9):795–8.

[13] Herth FJ, Eberhardt R, Vilmann P, et al. Real-time endobronchial ultrasound guided transbronchial needle aspiration for sampling mediastinal lymph nodes. Thorax 2006;61(9):795–8.

[14] Paone G, Nicastri E, Lucantoni G, et al. Endobronchial ultrasound-driven biopsy in the diagnosis of peripheral lung lesions. Chest 2005;128(5):3551–7.

[15] Herth FJ, Ernst A, Becker HD. Endobronchial ultrasound-guided transbronchial lung biopsy in solitary pulmonary nodules and peripheral lesions. Eur Respir J 2002;20(4):972–4.

[16] Herth FJ, Eberhardt R, Becker HD, et al. Endobronchial ultrasound-guided transbronchial lung biopsy in fluoroscopically invisible solitary pulmonary nodules: a prospective trial. Chest 2006;129(1): 147–50.

[17] Schwarz Y, Mehta AC, Ernst A, et al. Electromagnetic navigation during flexible bronchoscopy. Respiration 2003;70(5):516–22.

[18] Hautmann H, Schneider A, Pinkau T, et al. Electromagnetic catheter navigation during bronchoscopy: validation of a novel method by conventional fluoroscopy. Chest 2005;128(1):382–7.

[19] Schwarz Y, Greif J, Becker HD, et al. Real-time electromagnetic navigation bronchoscopy to peripheral lung lesions using overlaid CT images: the first human study. Chest 2006;129(4):988–94.

[20] Gildea TR, Mazzone PJ, Karnak D, et al. Electromagnetic navigation diagnostic bronchoscopy: a prospective study. Am J Respir Crit Care Med 2006;174(9):982–9.

**THORACIC
SURGERY
CLINICS**

ELSEVIER
SAUNDERS

Thorac Surg Clin 17 (2007) 167–173

Prognostic Modeling in Early Stage Lung Cancer: An Evolving Process from Histopathology to Genomics

David H. Harpole, Jr, MD

*Department of Surgery, Duke University Medical Center, Durham Veterans Affairs Medical Center,
DUMC Box 3627, Durham, NC 27710, USA*

Lung cancer is the leading cause of cancer death in the world. This disease was responsible for the deaths of 1.1 million people in 2000, representing about 18% of the total cancer deaths worldwide [1]. Pathologic stage I (75% of clinical stage I; >30,000 patients per year in North America) represents the fastest growing segment of patients with lung cancer because of the frequent use of high-resolution CT scans for screening. An estimated 60% 5-year survival is observed for these patients [2–4]. Four recent randomized phase III trials have demonstrated a survival advantage (4%–15%) for patients treated with adjuvant chemotherapy after resection in patients with pathologic stage II to IIIA [5–8], but data for adjuvant therapy in stage I are inconclusive [9], likely because of underpowered trials (an insufficient number of patients). A standard randomized trial including stage IA and IB may require randomization of more than 1000 patients to accumulate enough deaths for significant power to identify a real advantage for adjuvant cytotoxic chemotherapy. In addition, the likely benefit could be small compared with the risk encountered by stage I patients (up to 1% chemotherapy treatment-related mortality reported in previous trials and 60% do not need treatment). The goal is to validate a molecular-based tumor model that identifies patients at low-risk for cancer recurrence and who will not benefit from adjuvant chemotherapy. The remaining patients will be randomized to observation (present standard of care) or adjuvant chemotherapy to determine efficacy of adjuvant in this population.

Investigators at Duke University and others have focused on the identification of markers that may predict poor prognosis as a way to "enrich" the population by separating those likely to have early recurrence and cancer death from those not needing additional treatment after resection. Although aggressive tumors do not necessarily equate with tumors most likely to respond to a particular chemotherapy regimen, these high-risk patients have been the subset with the greatest benefit from adjuvant chemotherapy in most solid tumor systems (breast, colon, and so forth). The initial projects attempted to refine predictive models of cancer recurrence after resection for patients with early stage non–small cell lung cancer (NSCLC).

Histopathology and prognosis

A multitude of histopathologic factors were described in the literature from small, retrospective series that had an association with survival. This list was confusing; the author's laboratory undertook an investigation of all of these factors in a single, large cohort of NSCLC patients. Pathologic stage I was chosen to eliminate any interference from the powerful factors of distant and nodal metastases. No patients had adjuvant therapy after complete R0 resection. All tumors were recut and examined by a pulmonary pathologist for each factor blinded to outcome in a consecutive cohort of nearly 300 stage I patients after resection. Four factors were identified with an independent association with cancer-death (Table 1) [4].

E-mail address: harpo002@mc.duke.edu

1547-4127/07/$ - see front matter © 2007 Published by Elsevier Inc.
doi:10.1016/j.thorsurg.2007.03.014

thoracic.theclinics.com

Table 1

Multivariate Cox proportional hazards model of cancer death

Factor	Hazards ratio	P value
Pulmonary vascular invasion	2.36	.001
T2 tumor size	1.86	.002
Visceral pleural invasion	1.75	.022
>15 mitoses/HPF	1.51	.060

N = 289 stage I.

Protein expression and immunohistochemistry

Although observational data based on clinical and histopathologic description aided in dividing patients into risk group, much variation exists in interpretation of these qualitative variables. Improvement in molecular techniques has allowed refinements in predictive models. Investigations in the author's laboratory focused on protein expression measured with immunohistochemistry. Multiple algorithms could be created based on relative protein expression profiles using up to 15 factors with possible significance. Each of these factors with an independent association with survival represented a member of hypothetical groups created based on mechanism of action from a large cohort of pathologic stage I NSCLC who were followed for at least 5 years after resection and with no additional therapy (Table 2). Factors stained included cell cycle (rb, KI-67); apoptosis (p53, Bcl-2, Bax); tyrosine kinase growth factors (EGFr, Her2-neu); angiogenesis (factor VIII); basement membrane invasion (matrix metalloproteinase 9, UPA, UPAr); and cell adhesion-migration (E-selectin, CD-44, NCAM, blood group A) [10–16]. It is important to note that this model also was predictive for the 258 patients with stage IA disease, separating tumor into groups with a predicted 5-year survival ranging from 85% to 45% based on the number of these five factors expressed (0–5).

Table 2

Multivariate Cox proportional hazards model of cancer death

Factor	Hazards ratio	P value
p53	1.63	.0037
Angiogenesis (factor VIII)	1.47	.033
Her2-neu	1.43	.440
CD44	1.40	.050
Rb	0.747	.080

N = 408 stage I.

Although these models were effective in defining relative risk for patients with stage IA and IB NSCLC, individualized risk stratification was not possible. Lung cancer is a heterogeneous disease resulting from the acquisition of multiple somatic mutations; given this complexity, it would be surprising if a small set of gene or protein expression patterns could effectively describe and ultimately predict the clinical course of the disease for individual patients. The advent of near-genome-wide expression profiles has dramatically changed the field of molecular prognostics, however, and may allow for the potential of risk assessment for the individual. The challenge is recognizing and defining useful data from "noise" out of the thousands of simultaneous measurements. A new field of statistics, computation genomics, has developed novel methodology for successful completion of the task.

Building a novel genomic predictive model

A cohort of stage I patients was constructed with equal numbers of squamous cell carcinoma and adenocarcinoma, the histologies that constitute most NSCLC. Uniquely, equal numbers of patients with extremes of outcomes (good-risk tumors [those patients who lived >5 years after resection] and poor-risk tumors [those patients who died of metastatic cancer <2.5 years from resection]) were used to build the genomic model of tumor aggressiveness. The author's group has previously described methods to integrate multiple forms of data, including clinical variables and multiple gene expression profiles, to build robust predictive models for the individual patient [17–20]. There are several critical components to this methodologic approach. One must initially generate a collection of gene expression profiles (termed "metagenes"; an example of one metagene is shown in Fig. 1) that provide the basis for building the predictive models. These sets of 25 to 200 genes have the ability to separate the patients into survival cohorts. Next, these metagenes are grouped randomly to select those that are additive in predictive value (best predict the clinical outcome) using a regression tree analysis. An example tree (one of many generated in the analysis) is depicted in Fig. 1. The ultimate tree contained 100 branches and included over 2000 separate genes. A previously published gene expression-based model contained 30 to 540 genes in comparison [21–26].

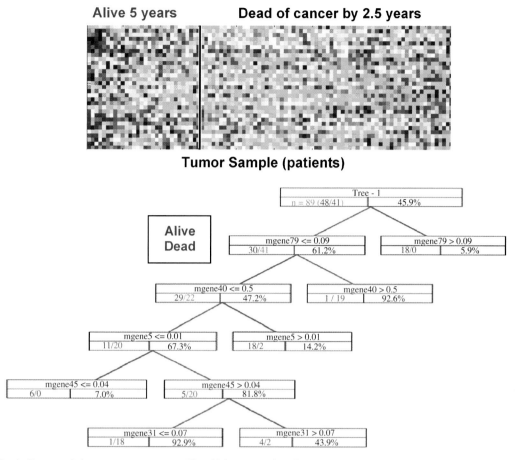

Fig. 1. Top panel demonstrates metagene 79, which separated patients into two survival groups. The bottom panel shows the first 5 of 100 steps in the tree that linked all of the metagenes that were identified as having additive power in separation of risk (red lines denote cancer death prediction).

Internal validation

The predictive accuracy of the metagene tree was assessed with various methods: internal validation (leave-one-out cross-validation and random test–training sets) and external validation (three separate non-Duke cohorts). Leave-one-out cross-validation is repeatedly performed; one sample is removed at each reanalysis and the recurrence probability is predicted for that one case. The entire model-building process is repeated for each prediction and evaluates the reproducibility of the approach. As shown in Fig. 2, the metagene-based model predicted recurrence with an overall accuracy of more than 90%. A 50% risk cut point was chosen for accuracy, sensitivity, and specificity. Next, as a measure of model stability, multiple iterations of randomly

split training and validation sets (two thirds of population as training set for the model and one third of population as a test set) from within the Duke cohort were generated and observed a greater than 85% accuracy in prognostic capability.

To compare these results to the clinical model, a similar process was used to create a "best" clinical model using the histopathologic variables defined in Table 1. The gene expression model for predicting recurrence was superior to a predictive clinical model generated. The c-statistic for the model with clinical variables was 0.65 and that for the genomic model greater than 0.9, adding strength to the conclusion that a gene expression–based prediction of outcome was superior to the current standard of care (using clinical variables). Even if the two models are combined,

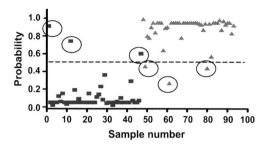

Fig. 2. The results of predictive model from gene array data (LMS, right panel) are demonstrated using the novel methodology and after a leave-one-out validation in the Duke Training Cohort. Individual risk was predicted for each tumor sample (patient). Orange triangles denote cancer death, and blue squares denote cure. The location along the y axis is the probability of cancer recurrence (death) predicted by the model. The accuracy was 94% and the sensitivity was 94%. The 6 of 91 errors of the gene array model are circled.

inclusion of the clinical data with the genomic data does not further improve the accuracy of the prediction of recurrence over the genomic data alone [27].

The samples used for the development of the genomic prognostic model represented equal numbers of both major histologic subtypes of NSCLC. The model was equally effective in predicting recurrence for both common histologic types (adenocarcinoma and squamous cell carcinoma), so it should be useful for most patients (Fig. 3).

The 2000-plus genes in this genomic prediction model (lung metagene score [LMS]) included several common oncogenic pathways (angiogenesis

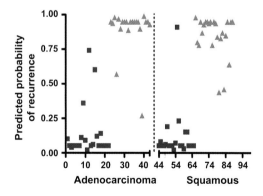

Fig. 3. The LMS works equally as well with adeno and squamous histology. Red triangles denote cancer death, and blue squares denote cure. The location along the y axis is the probability of cancer death predicted by the model.

[metagene 19], RAF, PI3kinase, and p53 signally pathway [metagene 41], among others).

External validation

Use of a prognostic model to assess risk of recurrence and to choose the appropriate use of adjuvant chemotherapy requires demonstration that the model is robust when applied to independent heterogeneous populations of patients and conditions of sample acquisition. Other investigators have developed predictive models for NSCLC, but little data are available that validate the models on external samples [21–26]. The author's group evaluated the ability of the model to predict recurrence risk using two multicenter cooperative group studies (American College of Surgeon Oncology Group [ACOSOG Z0030] and Cancer and Leukemia Group B [CALGB 9761]). These patients were resected and had fresh, frozen tumors collected in multiple CALGB and ACOSOG institutions. The patients were followed without adjuvant therapy. For all future investigations, a 50% probability of recurrence was defined as a cutoff for predicting recurrence.

A total of 25 samples were analyzed from the ACOSOG Z0030 trial. Eleven of 13 deaths were successfully predicted for an accuracy of 72% (sensitivity, 85%; specificity, 58%; positive predictive value, 69%; negative predictive value, 78%).

A total of 84 samples were analyzed from the CALGB 9761 trial as a second independent validation set. The outcome of these CALGB patients was blinded to the investigators applying the predictive model; the genomic predictions of recurrence were submitted to a CALGB statistician for a determination of outcome. The predictive accuracy of the model for the CALGB samples was 79% (sensitivity, 68%; specificity, 88%; positive predictive value, 79%; negative predictive value, 80%).

Finally, the metagene model was applied to another sample set of 15 patients with surgically resected stage I squamous cell lung cancer from another institution (Mayo Clinic). The model accurately predict the outcome in all five patients with recurrence, and 7 of 10 patients without recurrence, for an overall accuracy of 12 (80%) of 15 [27].

The planned trial will include stage IA and IB patients. Fig. 4 demonstrates the Kaplan-Meier survival plots for the 88 pathologic stage IA and IB patients from the three validation sets combined. The overall 5-year survival was 60% for these unselected patients. Note that patients with

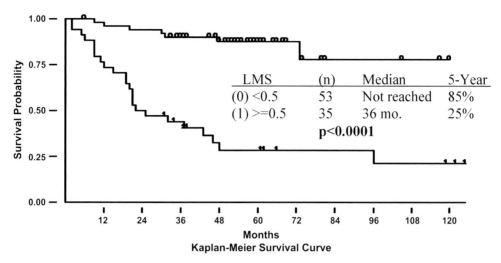

Fig. 4. Validation samples from ACOSOG Z0030, CALGB 9761, and Mayo Lung Bank. Note the hazards ratio for LMS ≥ 0.5 was 7.5. The tic marks are censored data.

a score greater than 0.5 ($\geq 50\%$ predicted death) had a 5-year survival of 25% (hazards ratio of 7.5) compared with the patients with a score less than 0.5 (survival 85% at 5 years). Interestingly, there were 60% low-score and 40% high-score patients, which matched the overall survival. These data are being used to power the adjuvant trial.

Future directions

The goal of the investigations over the last decade has been to refine prognosis as an opportunity to select patients for a prospective phase III adjuvant chemotherapy clinical trial. CALGB 30506, "A Randomized Phase III Trial to Evaluate the Lung Metagene Score to Direct Adjuvant Therapy in Stage 1 NSCLC Patients," is an intergroup-supported concept for a stage I NSCLC trial that uses the LMS to select appropriate patients for adjuvant therapy. The LMS is most accurate and specific for low-risk patients. It is being used to remove patients who do not need adjuvant therapy (low-score patients). The remaining patients (called intermediate-score patients) will be enrolled into a randomized adjuvant therapy treatment trial of observation (the present standard of care for pathologic stage I) versus adjuvant chemotherapy using the same chemotherapy doublets (cisplatin with docetaxel, vinorelbine, or gemcitabine) as the planned intergroup stage II to IIIA adjuvant therapy trial evaluating the efficacy of chemotherapy with or without

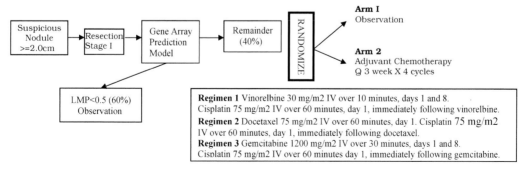

Fig. 5. CALGB 30506: an intergroup trial for stage I NSCLC patients using the LMS to select patients who are low score for observation (60% of total) and randomizing the rest (40%) for adjuvant therapy based on preference using the regimen from the new intergroup stage II-IIIA adjuvant trial (ECOG 1505). This trial is supported by NCI R01-CA 116648-01.

bevacizumab (Avastin) (ECOG 1505). The logistics of this trial have been defined and it is hoped that it may begin patient recruitment in 2007 (Fig. 5). This trial design represents a critical first step in the use of clinical genomics as a strategy to refine prognosis and improve the selection of patients appropriate for adjuvant chemotherapy.

References

[1] Parker SL, Tong T, Bolden S, et al. Cancer statistics. CA Cancer J Clin 1997;47(1):5–27.

[2] Naruke T, Goya T, Tsuchiya R, et al. Prognosis and survival in resected lung carcinoma based on the international staging system. J Thorac Cardiovasc Surg 1988;96:440–7.

[3] Strauss GM, Kwiatkowski DJ, Harpole DH Jr, et al. Molecular and pathologic analysis of stage I non-small cell lung carcinoma of the lung. J Clin Oncol 1995;13:1265–79.

[4] Harpole DH, Herndon JE, Young WG, et al. Stage I non-small cell lung cancer: a multivariate analysis of treatment and patterns of recurrence. Cancer 1995; 76:787–96.

[5] Kato H, Ichinose Y, Ohta M, et al. Japan Lung Cancer Research Group on Postsurgical Adjuvant Chemotherapy. A randomized trial of adjuvant chemotherapy with uracil-tegafur for adenocarcinoma of the lung. N Engl J Med 2004;350(17):1713–21.

[6] Arriagada R, Bergman B, Dunant A, et al. International Adjuvant Lung Cancer Trial Collaborative Group. Cisplatin-based adjuvant chemotherapy in patients with completely resected non-small-cell lung cancer. N Engl J Med 2004;350(4):351–60.

[7] Douillard J, Rosell R, Delena M, et al. ANITA: phase III adjuvant vinorelbine (N) and cisplatin (P) versus observation (OBS) in completely resected (stage I-III) non-small cell lung cancer (NSCLC) patients (pts): final results after 70-month median follow-up. Proceedings of the American Society of Clinical Oncology 2005; Abstract No 7013.

[8] Winton T, Livingston R, Johnson D, et al. Vinorelbine plus cisplatin vs. observation in resected non-small cell lung cancer. N Engl J Med 2005;352(25):2589–97.

[9] Strauss GM, Herndon JE, Maddaus MA, et al. Adjuvant chemotherapy in stage IB non-small cell lung cancer (NSCLC): update of Cancer and Leukemia Group B (CALGB) protocol 9633. Proceedings of the American Society of Clinical Oncology 2006; Abstract No. 7007.

[10] Harpole DH Jr, Herndon JE, Wolfe WG, et al. A prognostic model of recurrence and death in stage I non-small cell lung cancer utilizing presentation, histopathology, and oncoprotein expression. Cancer Res 1995;55:51–6.

[11] Harpole DH Jr, Marks JR, Richards W, et al. Localized adenocarcinoma of the lung: oncogene expression of erbB-2 and p53 in 150 patients. Clin Cancer Res 1995;1:659–64.

[12] Harpole DH Jr, Richards WG, Herdon JE, et al. Angiogenesis and molecular biologic sub-staging in patients with stage I non-small cell lung cancer. Ann Thorac Surg 1996;61:1470–6.

[13] Kwiatkowski DJ, Harpole DH Jr, Godleski J, et al. Molecular pathologic substaging in 244 STAGE I non-small cell lung cancer patients: clinical implications. J Clin Oncol 1998;16:2468–77.

[14] D'Amico TA, Massey M, Herndon JE II, et al. A biologic risk model for stage I lung cancer: immunohistochemical analysis of 408 patients using 10 molecular markers. J Thorac Cardiovasc Surg 1999; 117:736–43.

[15] D'Amico TA, Alioa TA, Herndon JE, et al. Molecular biologic sub-staging in patients with stage I non-small cell lung cancer: risk stratification according to sex and histological subtype. Ann Thorac Surg 2000;69:882–6.

[16] D'Amico TA, Moore MB, Aloia TA, et al. Predicting the site of metastases from lung cancer using molecular biologic markers. Ann Thorac Surg 2001;72: 1144–8.

[17] West M, Blanchette C, Dressman H, et al. Predicting the clinical status of human breast cancer by using gene expression profiles. Proc Natl Acad Sci USA 2001;98(20):11462–7.

[18] Pittman J, Huang E, Dressman H, et al. Models for individualized prediction of disease outcomes based on multiple gene expression patterns and clinical data. Proc Natl Acad Sci USA 2004;101: 8431–6.

[19] Pittman J, Huang E, Wang Q, et al. Bayesian analysis of binary prediction tree models for retrospectively sampled outcomes. Biostatistics 2004;5: 587–601.

[20] Nevins JR, Huang ES, Dressman H, et al. Towards integrated clinic-genomic models for personalized medicine: combining gene expression signatures and clinical factors in breast cancer outcomes prediction. Hum Mol Genet 2003;12:R153–7.

[21] Garber ME, Troyanskaya OG, Schluens K, et al. Diversity of gene expression in adenocarcinoma of the lung. Proc Natl Acad Sci USA 2001;98(24):13784–9.

[22] Bhattacharjee A, Richards WG, Staunton J, et al. Classification of human lung carcinomas by mRNA expression profiling reveals distinct adenocarcinoma subclasses. Proc Natl Acad Sci USA 2001;98(24): 13790–5.

[23] Beer DG, Kardia SL, Huang CC, et al. Gene-expression profiles predict survival of patients with lung adenocarcinoma. Nat Med 2002;8(8):816–24.

[24] Wigle DA, Jurisica I, Radulovich N, et al. Molecular profiling of non-small cell lung cancer and correlation with disease-free survival. Cancer Res 2002; 62(11):3005–8.

[25] Kikuchi T, Daigo Y, Katagiri T, et al. Expression profiles of non-small cell lung cancers on

cDNA microarrays: identification of genes for prediction of lymph-node metastasis and sensitivity to anti-cancer drugs. Oncogene 2003;22(14): 2192–205.

[26] Raponi M, Zhang Y, Yu J, et al. Gene expression signatures for predicting prognosis of squamous cell and adenocarcinomas of the lung. Cancer Res 2006;66(15):7466–72.

[27] Potti A, Mukherjee S, Prince R, et al. A genomic strategy to refine prognosis and therapeutic decision for adjuvant therapy in non-small cell lung carcinoma. N Engl J Med 2006;355(6):570–80.

ELSEVIER
SAUNDERS

Thorac Surg Clin 17 (2007) 175–190

THORACIC
SURGERY
CLINICS

Role of Sublobar Resection (Segmentectomy and Wedge Resection) in the Surgical Management of Non–Small Cell Lung Cancer

Brian L. Pettiford, MD*, Matthew J. Schuchert, MD,
Ricardo Santos, MD, Rodney J. Landreneau, MD

*Heart, Lung, and Esophageal Surgery Institute, Department of Surgery, University of Pittsburgh Medical Center,
Suite 715, Professional Office Building 1, UPMC Shadyside Medical Center,
5200 Centre Avenue, Pittsburgh, PA 15232, USA*

The use of sublobar resection as definitive management of resectable non–small cell lung cancer (NSCLC) has been a controversial topic throughout the history of surgery for lung cancer. Most thoracic surgeons continue to consider pulmonary resection less than lobectomy as inadequate for the management of lung cancers anatomically confined to a single lobe of the lung. Accordingly, sublobar resection is considered a compromise operation by many surgeons that should be used only for the management of small peripheral lung cancers present in patients with significant impairment in cardiopulmonary reserve, who cannot withstand the physiologic rigors of lobectomy.

The increasingly common finding of new subcentimeter malignant lesions identified through surveillance CT chest scanning efforts has led many surgeons to reassess the need for total lobectomy for the management of smaller peripheral NSCLC. In this setting a question frequently asked is, "Could anatomic segmentectomy or extended nonanatomic wedge resection be adequate for cure of the patient's lung cancer?" This article reviews the clinical information available today in formulating an opinion regarding the appropriate use of sublobar resection for the small peripherally located NSCLC. The technical details of the most commonly performed segmental resections are also described.

Historical perspective

Pulmonary segmentectomy was originally used for the resection of focal bronchiectasis and tuberculosis. Both of these pulmonary disease processes are commonly anatomically localized to discrete bronchopulmonary segments and the common bilateral involvement encourages the use of parenchymal-sparing resection techniques.

The first reported use of segmentectomy for the management of bronchiectasis is credited to Churchill and Belsey in 1939 [1]. Kent and Blades' [2] advocacy of individual ligation of bronchial and vascular hilar structures, coupled with Overholt and Langer's 1947 [3] description of the technique for resection of each bronchopulmonary segment in the treatment of bronchiectasis, established the use of anatomic segmentectomy for discrete sublobar pathology.

Interestingly, total pneumonectomy was still regarded as the only appropriate surgical option for the treatment of primary lung cancer during this period [4]. The dreadfully high mortality associated with pneumonectomy (40%) at that time led to the use of lobectomy as the preferred approach to resection of peripheral lung cancers [5].

The use of anatomic segmentectomy for the management of peripheral lung cancers was explored by some thoracic surgeons [6–9]; however, the relative complexity of the operative approach

---

* Corresponding author.
E-mail address: pettifordb@upmc.edu (B.L. Pettiford).

1547-4127/07/$ - see front matter © 2007 Elsevier Inc. All rights reserved.
doi:10.1016/j.thorsurg.2007.03.002

thoracic.theclinics.com

compared with lobectomy, and the increased morbidity related to prolonged air leak and local recurrence, deterred the enthusiasm of most surgeons for this approach to lung cancer [10]. The use of segmentectomy, and sublobar resection in general, was relegated as a compromise procedure for the management of patients with significant impairment in cardiopulmonary reserve having peripheral lung lesions confined within segmental anatomic boundaries [10–15].

An increasing body of evidence is emerging suggesting that sublobar resection with accurate nodal staging may be an adequate resection for small peripheral NSCLC. Surgical marginal status following sublobar resection continues to be an important concern and measures to enhance the marginal clearance continue to be explored [16–33].

Controversies regarding the use of segmentectomy

The use of anatomic segmentectomy is generally accepted for the management of benign disease processes and metastatic carcinoma to the lung confined to an anatomic segment. The use of sublobar resection and segmentectomy in particular has been accepted as a reasonable approach for resection in patients with significant impairment in cardiopulmonary reserve. The primary controversy over the years among thoracic surgeons has been with the use of segmentectomy as primary management of peripheral primary NSCLC for patients who are physiologically fit to undergo lobectomy.

This article reviews representative pertinent clinical investigations addressing the appropriateness of sublobar resection in the primary management of NSCLC. It must first be clarified that the authors believe sublobar resection is inappropriate for the management of most clinical NSCLC beyond that of stage I disease. For the most part, they favor the use of segmentectomy without adjuvant local therapy for small stage IA disease without endobronchial extension within anatomic segmental boundaries that are less than 2 cm in diameter (Fig. 1). Larger lesions are necessarily associated with anatomic margins of resection that are more prone to local recurrence unless adjuvant therapeutic measures to be discussed are considered (Figs. 2 and 3).

Is there compromise of patient survival with sublobar resection?

The argument of use of sublobar resection for stage I NSCLC attracted international attention with the initiation of the randomized trial of sublobar resection versus lobectomy for good-risk patients with stage IA disease conducted by the now defunct North American Lung Cancer Study Group during the late 1980s and early 1990s [11]. This study was inspired by the survival results seen among women undergoing less than total mastectomy for small primary breast cancers [34], and Erret's 1985 [35] reporting of equivalent survival results among stage I NSCLC patients with impaired cardiopulmonary reserve undergoing sublobar resection compared with physiologically fit stage I patients undergoing lobectomy.

The results of the Lung Cancer Study Group's efforts were reported in 1995 [11]. Primary findings of this study were that survival between sublobar resection and lobectomy were not significantly different, but local recurrence was three times greater when sublobar resection was

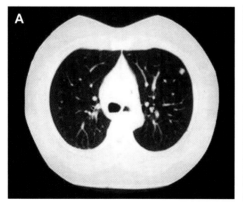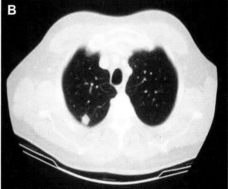

Fig. 1. (*A, B*) CT image of lesion ideal for sublobar resection (small peripheral T1 lesion confined to an anatomic segment).

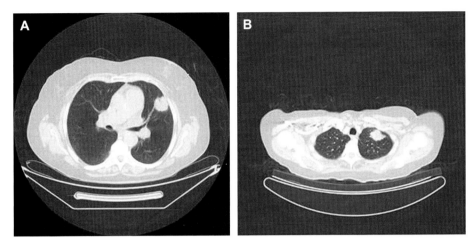

Fig. 2. (*A, B*) CT images of lesions for which adjuvant brachytherapy should be considered if sublobar resection is being performed. (T2 lesion confined to anatomic boundaries of the segment).

used. As an aside observation, they also stated that they found no difference in the loss of pulmonary functionality between lobectomy and sublobar resection patients when assessed 1 year following surgery. This important conclusion regarding postoperative functionality certainly caught the attention of many thoracic surgeons already convinced that lobectomy was the superior operation for even small stage I NSCLC. Interestingly, this conclusion regarding postoperative physiologic equivalency between resection approaches was made despite the fact that over one third of the patients in the study were not available for pulmonary function testing at the 1-year postoperative mark. Subsequent analyses of the late effects of relative pulmonary functional preservation with segmentectomy compared with lobectomy have countered the conclusions of this study [18,19]. Regardless of these findings, many thoracic surgeons continue to regard lobectomy as the gold standard treatment for early stage NSCLC.

In Japan, large CT radiologic screening programs in place for well over a decade have exposed an increased number of small, peripheral, early stage lung cancers [36]. Programs using fast CT scanners screening high-risk populations (older patients with significant smoking history and impairment in pulmonary function) are underway now in North America and Europe [37]. Renewed interests in sublobar resection and emerging enthusiasm with nonsurgical percutaneous management of small peripheral lung cancers identified through these efforts are now seen [18–25,29–32,38–41].

Interestingly, analyses that have compared sublobar resection with lobectomy identify patient age and the size of the tumor resected as the primary determinants of survival. Mery and colleagues [20] examined the effect of age and type of surgery on survival in patients with early-stage NSCLC. Their analysis of the Surveillance, Epidemiology, and End Results Database categorized the survival following resection of stage I NSCLC into three age groups: (1) less than 65 years, (2) 65 to 74 years, and (3) more than 75 years. A statistically greater number of elderly patients underwent

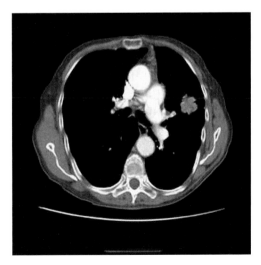

Fig. 3. Lesion for which lobectomy is required because of central lobar location limiting marginal clearance of the tumor.

limited resections, which included wedge resection. Two years following surgery, better survival was shown in young patients undergoing lobectomy as opposed to sublobar resection. No such survival time difference was demonstrated in the elderly population. Furthermore, the statistically significant long-term survival advantage favoring lobectomy for younger patients was lost compared with sublobar resection among patients greater than 70 years of age.

Okada and colleagues [21] conducted a retrospective analysis of 1272 consecutive patients who underwent complete resection with complete lymph node staging of NSCLC stratifying individuals in four groups according to tumor size: (1) 10 mm or less, (2) 11 to 20 mm, (3) 21 to 30 mm, and (4) more than 30 mm. The cancer-specific 5-year survivals were 100%, 83.5%, 76.5%, and 57.9%, respectively, for the four groups. Furthermore, no difference in cancer-specific survival was seen between patients undergoing lobectomy compared with segmentectomy for cancers smaller than 30 mm in diameter. The authors identified tumor size as an independent prognostic factor and suggested that segmentectomy with systematic nodal staging to avoid stage shift bias be considered as primary therapy for tumors 20 mm or less in size.

El-Sherif and colleagues [25] evaluated a 13-year experience in the management of resectable stage I NSCLC at their institution. The recurrence patterns and survival of 784 patients (577 lobectomies, 207 sublobar resections that were primarily wedges) who underwent resection of stage I NSCLC were evaluated. No significant differences were observed in disease-free survival between sublobar resection and lobectomy for patients with stage IA disease; however, a slightly worse disease-free survival was seen for stage IB patients undergoing sublobar resection compared with lobectomy (58% versus 50% 5-year disease-free survival). Sublobar resection was also associated with a lower overall 5-year survival compared with lobectomy (40% versus 54%) [16]. The authors suggested that this reduced overall survival following sublobar resection may have been related to the generally poorer functional status and comorbidities of the patients chosen for this resection rather than lobectomy at their institution.

Local recurrence concerns following sublobar resection

Although disease-free survival remains the most critical parameter in the assessment of any treatment-related modality for lung cancer, local recurrence following primary therapy is also an important concern. Local recurrence can result in significant morbidity, such as invasion into the chest wall or vital mediastinal structures, malignant pleural effusion, and problems related to airway obstruction and hemoptysis.

It is generally established that the risk of local recurrence is increased with the use of sublobar resection for the management of stage I NSCLC. Primary factors related to local recurrence are the surgical marginal distance of resection and the related presence of microscopic extension of disease or "in transit" local metastases. Inoue and colleagues [42] suggested that nodal involvement be considered in patients with lesions less than 2 cm diameter with pleural invasion or an elevated carcinoembryonic antigen level. Recent investigations have also noted that the molecular immunohistochemical assessment of the tissue margin may assist in predicting the risk for local recurrence following sublobar resection [17]. Such pathologic assessment of surgical margins may aid in decision-making regarding local adjuvant treatment measures or re-resection up to and including lobectomy to obtain disease clearance. The present recommendations for sublobar resection are to establish a margin at least that of the diameter of the pulmonary lesion resected [16].

Adjuvant radiotherapy has been considered as an option used in conjunction with sublobar resection possibly to reduce local recurrence. Miller and Hatcher [12] reported a significant decrease in local recurrence in follow-up of a small group of sublobar resection patients undergoing postoperative focal external beam "postage stamp" radiation compared with an earlier group of patients they managed with sublobar resection alone. Unfortunately, radiation treatment planning problems created by the unpredictable three-dimensional course of staple lines, the risk of local radiation injury to the treated remaining lobar segments of the lung, and the transportation difficulties associated with a several-week course of radiation therapy following thoracic surgery led to little enthusiasm with adjuvant external beam radiation therapy.

Others have used intraoperative brachytherapy as an adjunctive local control measure following lung resection associated with close or positive margins of resection. This use of adjuvant intraoperative brachytherapy was primary in the setting of locally advanced lung cancer where margins could not be reliably sterilized, and in an effort to provide immediate potential salvage therapy without the intrinsic delays associated with initiation of external beam radiotherapy after thoracotomy [26]. d'Amato and colleagues [27] were the first to report the use of intraoperative iodine 125 brachytherapy as a local measure following sublobar resection of peripheral stage I lung cancers when pathologically clear surgical margins had been obtained. These investigators described the fabrication of a radiation implant based on a polyglycolate hernia mesh template in which polyglycolate suture having iodine 125 pellets incorporated at 1-cm intervals along the length of the suture are woven into the mesh to create a treatment grid with pellets at 1-cm intervals (Fig. 4). This mesh template was then introduced into the chest and sutured onto the lung parenchymal surface at the suture line of resection to provide at least 2 cm of lateral margin coverage from the staple line. Usually 40 to 60 iodine 125 pellets within four to five lines of suture material were used with each brachytherapy implant. The total delivered radiation dose to the local tissues was calculated to be 10,000 cGY at a 1-cm depth. In essence, this very high intensity local therapy effectively extended the margin of resection by another centimeter. Santos and colleagues [28] subsequently reported a longitudinal follow-up of the use of intraoperative iodine 125 brachytherapy from the same institution, identifying that local

recurrence following sublobar resection seemed to be significantly reduced compared with historical control sublobar resection cases. On this further analysis, no local important radiation fibrosis, implant migration, or unexpected decline in postoperative pulmonary function was noticed among patients receiving intraoperative iodine 125 brachytherapy (Fig. 5).

Other retrospective reports of the use of intraoperative iodine 125 brachytherapy used with sublobar resection have been encouraging and have helped further to define the use of this adjuvant therapy approach aimed at reducing local recurrence. Fernando and associates [29] reported a retrospective multicenter analysis of 291 patients, which compared outcomes after lobectomy (N = 167) with those following sublobar resection (N = 124). Nearly one half of the sublobar resection group (N = 60) received adjuvant iodine 125 brachytherapy. The local recurrence rate in the sublobar resection group was decreased from 17.2% to 3.3% with the use of adjuvant iodine 125 brachytherapy. Finally, Birdas and colleagues [30] retrospectively compared the outcomes of sublobar resection with brachytherapy with lobectomy for patients with pathologic stage IB NSCLC. A total of 167 stage IB patients (126 patients undergoing lobectomy, 41 patients undergoing sublobar resection) were evaluated for local recurrence, disease-free survival, and overall survival. Local recurrence seen in the sublobar

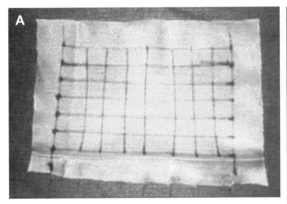
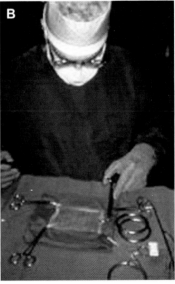

Fig. 4. Fabrication of brachytherapy implant. (*A*) Brachytherapy implant template. (*B*) Radiation oncologist fabricating radioactive iodine brachytherapy implant.

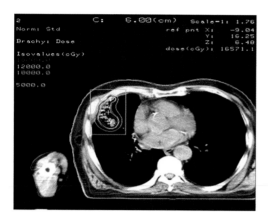

Fig. 5. Typical dosimetry calculation following brachy-therapy implant.

resection with iodine 125 brachytherapy group (4.8%) was similar to the lobectomy group (3.2%). There was no statistically significant difference in disease-free survival and overall survival between the two groups. These investigators concluded that sublobar resection with intraoperative iodine 125 brachytherapy provided equivalent local control, disease-free survival, and overall survival outcomes similar to lobectomy for IB NSCLC patients. In accordance with other investigators' concern for close surgical margins leading to increased risk for local recurrence [16], they emphasized the potential use of intraoperative iodine 125 brachytherapy in theoretically extending the margin of resection when larger (T2) tumors are chosen for sublobar resection.

Future investigative efforts regarding
the use of sublobar resection

Much of the information provided here has been the product of retrospective reviews of collected clinical experiences with sublobar resection. Randomized studies in progress or in conception will do much to define the role of sublobar resection and the use of adjuvant local control measures following these resections. Presently, the American College of Surgeons Oncology Group (ACOSOG) is conducting a randomized trial (Z04042) of sublobar resection (by anatomic segmentectomy or extended wedge resection) alone to similar sublobar resection with intraoperative iodine 125 brachytherapy for stage IA NSCLC. Over 200 patients are to be accrued for study. Cancer and Leukemia Group B is in the final phase of preparation of a randomized investigation of surgical resection of small (<2 cm in diameter) stage IA NSCLC by either lobectomy or sublobar resection by segmentectomy or wedge resection. Over 800 patients will be enrolled in this later study. The results of these studies should aid in establishing the role of sublobar resection in the future management of stage I NSCLC.

Preoperative evaluation before segmentectomy

Patients being considered for nonanatomic extended wedge resection or anatomic segmentectomy for the primary management of stage I NSCLC have usually been those with potentially important impairment in cardiopulmonary reserve. This may include borderline or marginal pulmonary functional physiology that prohibits formal lobectomy. Predicted postoperative pulmonary function based on the volume of functional pulmonary parenchyma to be resected may dictate the resection options for the patient with underlying pulmonary impairment.

Most patients present to the thoracic surgeon with an abnormal chest CT scan. This CT scan should include imaging of the liver and adrenal glands. Special attention should be focused on the mediastinum and the size and segmental location of the pulmonary parenchymal lesion in question. Mediastinoscopy is performed if indicated based on enlarged mediastinal lymph nodes (>1 cm in diameter) or fluorodeoxyglucose avidity on positron emission tomographic scanning. A complete pulmonary functional evaluation is indicated. This must include formal pulmonary spirometry, arterial blood gas analysis, and carbon monoxide diffusion capacity assessment. Split-lung ventilation-perfusion nuclear scintigraphic assessment and maximum oxygen consumption exercise testing may be selectively considered before surgery based on general functional concerns. Cardiac functional assessment using standard or pharmacologic stress testing and two-dimensional echocardiography with estimates of pulmonary arterial pressures should be considered. Radiation oncology consultation is obtained if adjuvant intraoperative iodine 125 brachytherapy is being considered as part of the treatment plan.

Operative techniques for anatomic pulmonary segmentectomy

Anesthetic airway control and thoracotomy incision

At the time of operation, laterality is marked. After intubation with a single-lumen endotracheal tube, a flexible bronchoscopy is performed in the standard fashion to ensure the absence of endobronchial extension of the malignant process precluding the use of sublobar resection. A double-lumen tube is then inserted and the patient positioned laterally. It is important that the thoracic surgeon confirm proper positioning of the endotracheal tube after initial placement and after patient lateral positioning to ensure the adequacy of selective contralateral lung ventilation and ipsilateral pulmonary atelectasis for the procedure. These actions can reduce the occurrence of time-consuming intraoperative problems associated with inadequate selective airway control with double-lumen intubation.

The authors prefer to use a vertical axillary muscle-sparing thoracotomy incision for most pulmonary resections [43]. During an upper lobe segmentectomy, the incision is placed at the lower border of the axillary hairline in the mid-axillary plane, and extended distally for 8 cm (Fig. 6). The pectoralis minor muscle is reflected anteriorly. The muscle fibers of the serratus anterior muscle

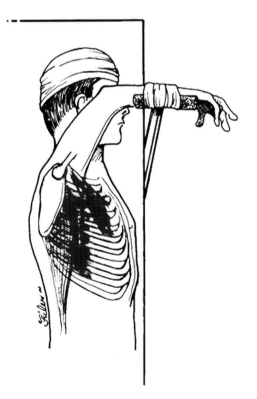

Fig. 6. Vertical axillary incisions for upper and lower sublobar resection. Note the incision location relative to the serratus anterior, pectoralis minor, and latissimus dorsi muscles.

lying over the third rib are split. The lateral aspect of the third rib is resected subperiosteally and a 2-cm portion of the fourth rib is also resected to enhance further mini thoracotomy exposure. Two pediatric rib spreaders are inserted and positioned at right angles to each other for exposure.

For lower lobe segmental resections, the skin incision is begun approximately 3 cm inferior to the axillary hairline along the posterior axillary line, near the anterior border of the latissimus dorsi muscle and a similar 8-cm incisional length used for thoracotomy. The latissimus dorsi is reflected posteriorly and the serratus anterior is detached along a segment of its inferior muscular origin. The fourth rib is resected subperiosteally, and a 2-cm portion of the fifth rib is removed. The authors have found that these vertical approaches allow for adequate exposure through a mini thoracotomy incision with minimal chest wall trauma [44]. This vertical incision approach also increases versatility in accessing a number of segments of the lung, and it is relatively cosmetically appealing compared with lateral thoracotomy.

Primary bronchopulmonary segmental anatomy

In normal pulmonary anatomy, the right and left lungs are comprised of 19 bronchopulmonary segments. A total of 10 segments constitute the right lung and nine contribute to the left lung. A pulmonary segment consists of a sublobar bronchovascular unit and the corresponding pulmonary parenchyma that it serves. Anatomic segmentectomy refers to the removal of one or more pulmonary parenchymal segments and the corresponding bronchovascular supply. A nonanatomic or wedge resection refers to sublobar resection without isolation and removal of the bronchovascular unit supplying the targeted lung parenchyma.

Anatomic variation in the volume of the segmental anatomy of each lobe of the lung is not uncommon. This variation may be congenital in nature or a result of parenchymal changes from the primary lung pathology or the induction therapies used before resection. When evaluating the possibility of segmentectomy or bisegmentectomy for a pulmonary lesion resection, it is critical to ensure that the remaining or residual segment of the lobe is of adequate functional size to merit the decision to perform the sublobar resection.

Apical and apicoposterior segmentectomy

The apical segment may be resected alone or in combination with the posterior segment as a formal apicoposterior segmentectomy. During apical segmentectomy, the anterior hilar pleural envelope is opened using electrocautery or dissecting scissors. Special care is taken to avoid injury to the phrenic nerve pedicle located medial to the pulmonary hilum. The apical segmental vein from the superior branch of the right upper lobe vein is isolated as it crosses the right upper lobe pulmonary artery. Blunt dissection about the bronchovascular hilar structures using either a "peanut" dissector or the tip of a pediatric metal Yankauer suction device is primarily performed. Electrocautery and scissor division of areolar tissues are accomplished as necessary. A right angle forceps is passed around the segmental vein and then encircled with a 0-silk tie. An endostapler for pulmonary vascular ligation is introduced through a trocar located at a lower intercostal access that is used for subsequent chest tube introduction. The vessel is then divided using the endostapler with a 2.5 mm in height (vascular) staple load or it can be alternatively ligated with 0-silk sutures (Fig. 7). This maneuver exposes the underlying superior division of the right pulmonary artery, including the apical and anterior branches. The apical segmental branch is the more superior of the two vessels. The perivascular plane is entered and the apical segmental artery is exposed. A right angle forceps is used to create an adequate space for the future endostapler application. The vessel is isolated and divided as described previously for division of the segmental vein. The parietal pleura is then incised along the superior hilum and extended posteriorly inferior to the azygous vein to the upper edge of the right upper lobe bronchus when right-sided resections are performed. The inferior aspect of the aortic arch at the aorticopulmonary artery window is the anatomic boundary during left-sided resections. The apical segment bronchus is exposed by gently sweeping the peribronchial

pulmonary parenchyma away from the bronchial stump toward segmental lung tissue to be resected. If the anatomic distinction of the correct segmental bronchus for resection is in doubt, it is prudent to clamp the segmental bronchus followed by lung ventilation to confirm atelectasis of the proposed segment to be resected. The apical bronchus is then divided as described previously for vascular interruption. A 3.5-mm height staple load of the endostapler is used for segmental bronchial staple closure and simultaneous division. The specimen side of the transected bronchus is then grasped with an Allis clamp to delineate and secure the proximal base of the pulmonary segment within the resected specimen (Fig. 8). The segmentectomy is completed using multiple firings of a 45-mm endostapler with 3.5 mm and 4.8 mm in height stapler loads depending on the thickness of the pulmonary parenchymal line of resection. The authors prefer to use an endostapler in lieu of the standard GIA or TA instruments to staple and transect the pulmonary parenchyma and bronchus because of the ability to introduce the endostapler through an accessory intercostal access site and avoid a larger primary thoracotomy incision necessary to introduce the standard stapling devices [44].

Some view this parenchyma stapling technique as potentially distorting to the remaining lung, and a significant risk to the venous drainage of the adjacent segment of the lobe through the common intersegmental venous anatomy. This theoretical concern has not been a clinical problem when

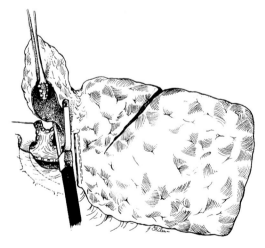

Fig. 8. Apical segmentectomy. An Allis clamp is elevating the specimen side of the transected bronchus. This serves as a base for the parenchymal division.

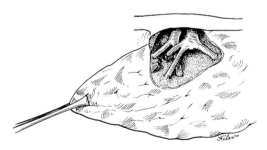

Fig. 7. Anterior hilar dissection with ligation of apical segmental venous branch.

a single segment of a lobe is resected. The authors are aware of this potential drainage problem when a bisegmentectomy is performed. Collateral venous drainage through the remaining segmental venous system is reliable so as to avert parenchymal dysfunction or important venous congestion. The primary advantage of this stapled resection approach is the potential reduction in bleeding and bronchopleural fistula from the raw surface of the residual segment's surface when the "finger fracture" technique of dissection along the intersegmental venous boundaries is used. Bronchopleural fistula and air leak associated with this latter approach can be significant and prolonged leading to extension in hospitalization, pulmonary space problems, and empyema.

On completion of the endostapler segmental resection, it is critically important to ensure that segmental bronchial closure is secure and that the staple line of parenchymal resection has minimal, if any, air leak. The use of staple line bolstering material or topical sealants may be helpful in obtaining pneumonstasis when the pulmonary parenchyma is emphysematous or indurated [45,46].

Posterior segmentectomy

Right upper lobe posterior segmentectomy is readily accomplished by initially approaching the superior posterior aspect of the pulmonary hilum to identify the right upper lobe bronchus. The superior hilar pleural lining is incised and the right upper lobe bronchus exposed using blunt dissection. The posterior segmental bronchus is best approached posteriorly and isolated by sweeping the overlying lung parenchyma distally. The bronchus is carefully encircled using a blunt right angle forceps. Special care is taken to avoid injury to the posterior segmental artery, which lies immediately anterior to the bronchus from this posterior vantage point during the dissection about the segmental bronchus. This may be minimized by carefully dissecting between the bronchus and artery using a blunt dissector. A 0-silk tie is used to encircle the bronchus, and blunt dissection is used to create a plane to accommodate the endostapler. The bronchus is divided with a 3.5-mm staple load (Fig. 9). The posterior segmental artery is then isolated similarly and divided using a 2.5-mm vascular load of the endostapler. The specimen side of the segmental bronchus is secured using an Allis clamp, and the parenchymal margin of resection as

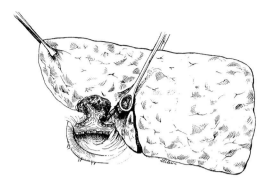

Fig. 9. Division of posterior segmental bronchus. The posterior segmental artery lies deep to the transected bronchus and is intimately located along the anterior aspect of the segmental bronchus.

described for apical segmentectomy (Fig. 10). In this case, the segmental pulmonary venous drainage to the posterior segment is often seen as several terminal arboration of the interlobar pulmonary vein. Hemoclip ligation and division of these smaller branches can be readily performed before stapler ligation of the parenchyma at the segmental margin.

An alternative approach may be taken in patients with a completely developed posterior aspect of the major fissure where exposure of the interlobar pulmonary artery is relatively straightforward. The interlobar pulmonary artery is exposed in the standard fashion by entering the perivascular sheath. The superior segmental and the right middle lobe arteries are identified during

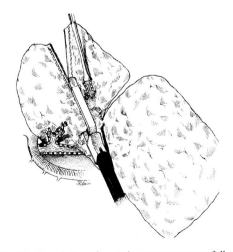

Fig. 10. Completion of posterior segmentectomy following bronchovascular division.

the course of right-sided resections. Rarely, the posterior segmental artery may arise from the superior segmental artery, particularly if the latter vessel originates as a large trunk. More often, dissection along the interlobar right pulmonary artery identifies the posterior segmental artery, which arises anteriorly at a right angle to the origin of the superior segmental artery beyond the middle lobe segmental arteries. Once identified, the posterior segmental artery is isolated and divided. The authors generally avoid this approach in patients with incompletely developed posterior major fissures to avoid unnecessary parenchymal bleeding and air leak.

During left side posterior segmental resections, the primary concern following establishment of the interlobar plane and identification of the interlobar pulmonary artery is avoiding the division of high lingular arterial branches, which may be confused as accessory posterior segmental vasculature. After division of the posterior segmental artery or arteries, the posterior segmental bronchus can be palpated with blunt dissection. During the dissection of the left posterior segmental bronchus it is important to avoid injury to the closely apposed venous drainage of the segment and the anterior and apical pulmonary segmental arteries anterior to it. Allis clamp is used to grasp the bronchial stump and the parenchymal margin of resection established with the 45-mm endostapler, with the bronchial stump maintained at the base of the resection.

Anterior segmentectomy of the right upper lobe

Right upper lobe anterior segmentectomy is the most technically difficult segmental resection to master. The anatomic location of the anterior segmental bronchus is not readily accessible by the anterior pulmonary hilum because the segmental vasculature to the apical segment of the upper lobe is more superficially located. The apical segmental vasculature must necessarily be "worked around" during the dissection of the deeper anterior segmental bronchopulmonary anatomy.

The mediastinal pleural lining over the anterior pulmonary hilum is incised, as for apical segmentectomy. The authors find it useful to divide the horizontal fissure separating middle from upper lobes at this point to reveal the interlobar extension of the upper lobe vein and the inferior aspect of the anterior segment of the upper lobe. The superior pulmonary vein branch of the upper lobe

vein is then exposed by sharp and blunt dissection. The apical segmental vein is identified as it crosses the truncus anterior of the right pulmonary artery. The apical and anterior veins are noted to converge to form the upper trunk of the superior pulmonary vein. The anterior segmental vein is the more inferior and deeply located of the two vessels. This vessel is isolated and divided with an endostapler or between 0-silk ties using an extracorporeal tying technique (Fig. 11). Beneath the apical segmental vein branch, the superior trunk of the right pulmonary artery is dissected peripherally, exposing the apical and anterior segmental arterial branches. The more inferiorly located anterior branch is isolated and divided (Fig. 11A). The interlobar pulmonary vein is gently reflected inferiorly, and the anterior segmental arterial stump and apical segmental vein reflected superiorly to expose the anterior segmental bronchus. Small venous tributaries are often encountered leading to the interlobar upper lobe vein, which must be individually ligated and divided. The anterior segmental bronchus can then be encircled with a right-angled forceps and divided using an endostapler with a 3.5-mm staple load (Fig. 11B). The anterior segmental bronchus is grasped and the parenchymal margin of resection determined as previously described by partial inflation of the lung to demarcate the zone of anterior segment atelectasis and inflation of the apical and posterior segments. The parenchymal resection then ensues using a 45-mm endostapler device.

Superior segmentectomy

The approach to superior segmentectomy begins with identification of the interlobar pulmonary artery in the major fissure. When the major

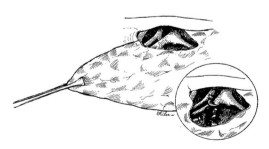

Fig. 11. Anterior segmentectomy showing the hilar vascular relationship. Division of the anterior segmental artery and vein provides access to the anterior segmental bronchus.

fissure is incomplete, it is sometimes necessary to estimate the line of demarcation between the upper and lower lobes and use the 45-mm endo-stapler to divide the pulmonary parenchyma along this line. The authors prefer this approach to blind sharp or electrocautery excavation of the fissure at the mid point, or "sump zone," of the pulmonary hilum between the upper and lower lobes. This maneuver can be done from posteri-orly between the posterior segment of the upper lobe and superior segment of the lower lobe or from an anterior inferior location by dividing the parenchymal connection between the basilar seg-ments and the lateral segment of the middle lobe. Once the interlobar pulmonary artery is exposed, the perivascular plane is entered. Posterior dissec-tion along the course of the interlobar artery identifies the superior segmental artery inferiorly.

On the right, a lateral segmental branch of right middle lobe artery is commonly seen medi-ally and proximal to the origin of the superior segmental artery. The posterior segmental artery is identified slightly proximal and opposite the superior segmental artery on the axis of the interlobar pulmonary artery. Occasionally, the posterior segmental artery arises from the supe-rior segmental artery. It is obviously important to ligate distal to the posterior segmental vessel artery from this common trunk. The superior segmental artery is isolated and divided.

When approaching the left lower lobe superior segment, the anatomic relationships are somewhat different. The superior segmental artery is identi-fied posteriorly along the axis of the interlobar artery opposite the more anterior position of the posterior segmental artery branch of the left upper lobe.

The relationship of the superior segmental bronchus to the superior segmental artery is similar bilaterally. The superior segmental bron-chus can be palpated and visualized with minimal dissection deep to the transected superior segmen-tal arterial stump (Fig. 12). Encirclement and divi-sion of the superior segmental bronchus is accomplished as mentioned previously. The supe-rior segmental vein, which lies just posterior and inferior to the segmental bronchus, may be in-jured if the bronchus is not encircled closely and carefully. The parenchymal resection of the seg-mentectomy is completed using the specimen side of the bronchus as a handle while dividing the parenchyma with a 45-mm endostapler, along the margin of atelectasis between it and the basilar segments of the lower lobe.

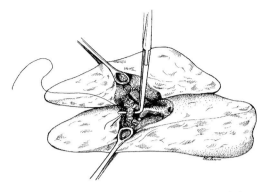

Fig. 12. Right superior segmentectomy performed along the oblique fissure. Note that the bronchus lies posterior to the segmental artery when approached through the oblique fissure.

Basilar segmentectomy

When one speaks of basilar segmentectomy, it is describing the resection of all four basilar segments of the lower lobe as a single unit. In many respects, performance of the dissection for a basilar segmentectomy is the mirror image of the dissection for superior segmentectomy. The key issue in performance of a basilar segmentectomy is the identification and preservation of the superior segmental vein during the dissection of the basilar segmental vein. The first maneuver is to divide the inferior pulmonary ligament to delineate the inferior aspect of the pulmonary hilum and the detail of the inferior pulmonary vein. The basilar segmental vein is usually a large trunk with a primary bifurcation between it and the superior segmental vein. This relationship is established and the basilar segmental venous trunk ligated and divided with a 2.5-mm vascular load of the endostapler. The parenchymal bridge of the lower aspect of the major fissure between middle lobe on the right or the lingular segment of the upper lobe on the left and the basilar segments of either lobe is now divided with the endostapler. This exposes the basilar segmental artery in the interlobar hilar plane. The middle lobe artery and lingular segmental artery depending on the side of resection are identified proximal and anterior to the main basilar arterial trunk. The superior segmental artery of either lower lobe is usually noted proximal and posterior along the course of the interlobar artery as it is dissected from the lower aspect of the main basilar arterial trunk. After division of the basilar segmental arterial trunk with the 2.5-mm vascular of the endostapler, the basilar segmental bronchus is palpable beneath the stump of the interlobar pulmonary artery. Blunt dissection delineates the bifurcation with the superior segmental bronchus and the basilar segmental bronchus to be transected. The basilar bronchus is encircled and before its ligation clamped to reinflate the lung and ensure that the superior segmental bronchus has not been inadvertently included in the bronchial encirclement. After aeration of the superior segment is ensured, the basilar segmental bronchus is ligated and divided with the 3.5-mm load of the endostapler. The specimen side of the bronchus is grasped with an Allis clamp and the parenchymal margin of resection accomplished with the 45-mm endostapler as described previously.

Left upper lobe upper division segmentectomy

An upper division segmentectomy of the left upper lobe is sometimes referred to as a "lingular-sparing" left upper lobectomy. The authors continue to include this resection within the concept of segmental lung resection, as is the description of left upper lobe lingulectomy that follows.

The pleural lining over the upper lobe vein is incised and the bifurcation between the superior branch of the upper lobe vein and the lingular vein is identified. The superior branch of the upper lobe vein is encircled and transected with the 2.5-mm load of the endostapler. The pulmonary arterial branches to the anterior segment and apical segment of the upper lobe are now identified along the superior arch of the pulmonary artery and these can usually be isolated with minimal dissection unless peribronchial lymphadenopathy is present. These vessels may originate as a common trunk. After division of these vessels with the 2.5-mm load of the endostapler, the upper division bronchus can be palpated and bluntly dissected to establish the bifurcation with the lingular bronchus at this point when dissecting from an anterior plane of orientation. The upper aspect of the major fissure is completed if necessary with endostapler application to separate the posterior segment of the upper lobe from the superior segment of the lower lobe. This exposes the posterior segmental arterial supply, which can be multiple.

The arterial anatomy to the left upper lobe is the most variable of all lobes of the lungs. Attention to this detail can avoid inadvertent injury to remaining segmental vessels intact at the incorrect perception of completion of the dissection by the surgeon. When dissecting about the superior aspect of the left pulmonary hilum, it is also important to stay within the perivascular plane to avoid possible injury to the left recurrent laryngeal nerve located beneath the aortic arch in the aorticopulmonary window.

The posterior segmental artery or arteries are ligated and divided. After this has been accomplished, a relatively easy completion of the tunnel between the anterior and the interlobar aspect of the pulmonary hilum can be established at the bifurcation of upper division and lingular bronchi of the upper lobe. The upper division bronchus is encircled and temporarily occluded and the left lung is expanded temporarily. This maneuver insures patency of the lingular bronchus and aeration of the lingular segment. The upper division bronchus is divided with the 3.5-mm load of the endostapler and the parenchymal margin determined by the zone of atelectasis between the upper division segment and the previously aerated lingular segment. The parenchymal resection is performed with the 45-mm endostapler.

Lingulectomy

During lingulectomy, the mediastinal pleural lining is incised along the anterior left hilum. The lingular vein is identified as the lower tributary of the upper lobe pulmonary vein. The lingular bronchus can now be palpated beneath the stump of the lingular vein and anterior blunt dissection can establish the bifurcation with the upper division bronchus of the upper lobe. Dissection along the inferior aspect of the anterior pulmonary hilum can also establish the division between the lower aspect of the upper lobe vein and the lower lobe venous trunk. Appreciation of this anatomic relationship is important as one proceeds to division of the parenchymal bridge of lung tissue that may exist between the inferior lingular segment and the basilar segments of the lower lobe. This parenchymal bridge is divided using the endostapler to identify the basilar segmental artery posteriorly and the lingular segmental pulmonary artery anteriorly at the interlobar zone of the pulmonary hilum. The interlobar pulmonary artery is then exposed within this interlobar zone of the major fissure. There may be more than one lingular arterial branch and these must be divided taking care to avoid inadvertent ligation of the more superiorly located posterior segmental pulmonary artery or arteries (Fig. 13). The interlobar pulmonary artery

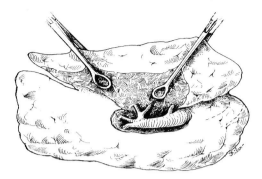

Fig. 13. Interlobar exposure of the left pulmonary artery. In this horizontal orientation, the vertically positioned hilar vessels depicted are the lingular and posterior segmental branches, respectively.

is then reflected laterally and completion of the dissection about the lingular bronchus accomplished. The bronchus is encircled and clamped. The lung is expanded to ensure that the upper division bronchus is patent and the upper division aerated. The lingular bronchus is then transected with the 3.5-mm load of the endostapler and the parenchymal margin of resection accomplished as described previously (Figs. 14 and 15).

Intraoperative brachytherapy

To reduce the likelihood of local recurrence, the authors commonly use adjuvant iodine 125 brachytherapy in patients where they have performed anatomic segmentectomy or extended wedge resections as definitive management of NSCLC. The authors conform to the technical details for creation of the brachytherapy implant and insertion described previously by d'Amato and colleagues [27]. An alternative approach described by Lee and colleagues [47] involves direct suturing of the polyglycolic acid suture with the incorporated

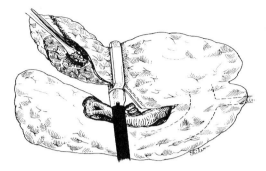

Fig. 15. Parenchymal division during lingulectomy with preservation of the basilar segmental bronchus and upper division parenchyma.

iodine 125 pellets within its length directly to the lung surface without the use of the polyglycolic acid hernia mesh template. The relative merits of these approaches are one of the points of analysis in the ACOSOG Z04032 study mentioned previously.

Thoracoscopic approach to formal segmentectomy

The video-assisted thoracoscopic surgical approach for segmental resections is similar to that for video-assisted thoracoscopic surgical lobectomy (Fig. 16). The performance of video-assisted thoracoscopic surgical segmentectomy does add a new dimension to the hilar dissection that is not appreciated with video-assisted thoracoscopic surgical lobectomy. The details of the dissection are basically the same as that described here for

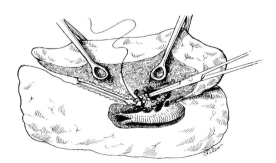

Fig. 14. Parenchymal division during lingulectomy with elevation of the lingular bronchovascular pedicle.

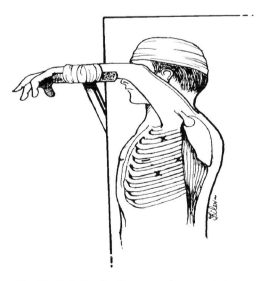

Fig. 16. Port sites for thoracoscopic segmentectomy.

segmentectomy performed through a mini muscle-sparing thoracotomy. Shiraishi and colleagues [48] demonstrated the feasibility of thoracoscopic segmentectomy and complete hilar and mediastinal lymph node dissection. They outlined clinical indications for video-assisted thoracoscopic surgical segmentectomy that include the following: small, peripheral lesions less than 2 cm; no lymph node or intrapulmonary metastases as suggested by high-resolution CT; and a 2-cm margin between the tumor and the segmental margin. The application of a brachytherapy implant is also easily accomplished with the video-assisted thoracoscopic surgical approach when this adjuvant measure is believed to be an important compliment for local control of the lung cancer [27].

Summary

Segmentectomy demands a thorough knowledge of the three-dimensional bronchovascular anatomy of the lung. This anatomic detail makes segmentectomy significantly more challenging than lobectomy. Several principles must be applied when performing segmental lung resection: (1) the surgeon should avoid dissection in a poorly developed fissure, (2) use the transected bronchus as the base of the segmental resection during the division of the lung parenchymal in the intersegmental plane, (3) consider the use of endostapler division of the pulmonary parenchyma to reduce the air leak complications related to "finger fracture" dissection of the intersegmental plane, and (4) consider the use of adjuvant iodine 125 brachytherapy as a means of reducing local recurrence following sublobar resection.

Increasing evidence supports the use of anatomic segmentectomy in the treatment of primary lung cancer for appropriately selected patients. This resection approach seems most appropriate in the management of the small (<2 cm in diameter) peripheral stage I NSCLC in which a generous margin of resection can be obtained. Accurate intraoperative nodal staging is important to estimate the relative use of these approaches compared with more aggressive resection and to determine the need for adjuvant systemic therapy if metastatic lymphadenopathy is identified. Future investigations comparing the results of sublobar resection with lobectomy will more clearly define the role of segmentectomy among good-risk patients with clinical stage I NSCLC. At the present time, it seems that

sublobar resection is an appropriate therapy for the management of stage I NSCLC identified in the elderly patient, those individuals with significant cardiopulmonary dysfunction, and for the management of peripheral solitary metastatic disease to the lung. Because the primary disadvantage of sublobar resection is that of local recurrence, intraoperative adjuvant iodine 125 brachytherapy may be considered to minimize this local recurrence risk.

Acknowledgments

The authors acknowledge the service of Mr. Ron Filer in the creation of the drawings. Mr. Filer is affiliated with the Medical Media Services of the University of Pittsburgh Medical Center.

References

[1] Churchill ED, Belsey R. Segmental pneumonectomy in bronchiectasis. Ann Surg 1939;109:481–99.
[2] Kent EM, Blades B. The anatomic approach to pulmonary resection. Ann Surg 1942;116:782.
[3] Overholt RH, Langer L. A new technique for pulmonary segmental resection, its application in the treatment of bronchiectasis. Surg Gynecol Obstet 1947;84:257–68.
[4] Oschner A, DeBakey M. Primary pulmonary malignancy: treatment by total pneumonectomy. Analysis of 79 collected cases and presentation of 7 personal cases. Surg Gynecol Obstet 1939;68:435–41.
[5] Churchill ED, Sweet RH, Sutter L, et al. The surgical management of carcinoma of the lung: a study of cases treated at the Massachusetts General Hospital from 1930–50. J Thorac Cardiovasc Surg 1950;20:349–65.
[6] Churchill ED, Sweet RH, Souter L, et al. Further studies in the surgical management of carcinoma of the lung. J Thorac Surg 1958;36:301–8.
[7] Bonfils-Roberts EA, Clagett OT. Contemporary indication for pulmonary segmental resections. J Thorac Surg 1972;63:433–8.
[8] Jensik RJ, Faber LP, Milloy FJ, et al. Segmental resection for a lung cancer: a fifteen year experience. J Thorac Cardiovasc Surg 1973;66:563–72.
[9] Read RC, Yoder G, Schaeffer RC. Survival after conservative resection for TINOMO non-small cell lung cancer. Ann Thorac Surg 1990;49:242–7.
[10] Warren WH, Faber LP. Segmentectomy versus lobectomy in patients with stage I pulmonary carcinoma. J Thorac Cardiovasc Surg 1994;107:1087–94.
[11] Ginsberg RJ, Rubenstein LV for the Lung Cancer Study Group. Randomized trial of lobectomy vs. limited resection for TINO non-small cell lung cancer. Ann Thorac Surg 1995;60:615–23.

[12] Miller JI, Hatcher CR. Limited resection of bronchogenic carcinoma in the patient with marked impairment of pulmonary function. Ann Thorac Surg 1987;44:340–3.

[13] Landreneau RJ, Sugarbaker DJ, Mack MJ, et al. Wedge resection versus lobectomy for stage I (T1N0M0) non-small cell lung cancer. J Thorac Cardiovasc Surg 1997;113(4):691–700.

[14] Shennib H, Landreneau RJ, Mack MJ. Video assisted thoracoscopic wedge resection of T1 lung cancer in high risk patients. Ann Surg 1993;218:555–60.

[15] Lewis RJ. The role of video-assisted thoracic surgery for carcinoma of the lung: wedge resection to lobectomy by simultaneous individual stapling. Ann Thorac Surg 1993;56:762–8.

[16] Sawabata N, Ohta M, Matsumura A, et al. Thoracic Surgery Study Group of Osaka University. Optimal distance of malignant negative margin in excision of nonsmall cell lung cancer: a multicenter prospective study. Ann Thorac Surg 2004;77(2):415–20.

[17] Masasyesva BG, Tong BC, Brock MV, et al. Molecular margin analysis predicts local recurrence after sublobar resection of lung cancer. Int J Cancer 2005;113(6):1022–5.

[18] Keenan RJ, Landreneau RJ, Maley RH Jr, et al. Segmental resection spares pulmonary function in patients with stage I lung cancer. Ann Thorac Surg 2004;78(1):228–33.

[19] Harada H, Okada M, Sakamoto T, et al. Functional advantage after radical segmentectomy versus lobectomy for lung cancer. Ann Thorac Surg 2005;80:2041–5.

[20] Mery CM, Pappas AN, Bueno R, et al. Similar long-term survival of elderly patients with non-small cell lung cancer treated with lobectomy or wedge resection within the surveillance, epidemiology, and end results database. Chest 2005;128(1):13–4.

[21] Okada M, Nishio W, Sakamoto T, et al. Effect of tumor size on prognosis in patients with non-small cell lung cancer: the role of segmentectomy as a type of lesser resection. J Thorac Cardiovasc Surg 2005;129(1):87–93.

[22] Yoshikawa K, Tsubota N, Kodama K, et al. Prospective study of extended segmentectomy for small lung tumors: the final report. Ann Thorac Surg 2002;73:1055–9.

[23] Koike T, Yamato Y, Yoshiya K, et al. Intentional limited pulmonary resection for peripheral T1N0M0 small-sized lung cancer. J Thorac Cardiovasc Surg 2003;125:424–928.

[24] Okada M, Yoshikawa K, Hatta T, et al. Is segmentectomy with lymph node assessment an alternative to lobectomy for non-small cell lung cancer of 2 cm or smaller? Ann Thorac Surg 2001;71:956–61.

[25] El-Sherif A, Santos R, et al. Outcomes of sublobar resection versus lobectomy for stage I non-small cell lung cancer: a 13-year analysis. Ann Thorac Surg 2006;82:408–16.

[26] Nori D, Li X, Pugkhem T. Intraoperative brachytherapy using Gelfoam radioactive implants for resected stage III non-small cell lung cancer with positive margin: a pilot study. J Surg Oncol 1995;60:257–61.

[27] d'Amato TA, Galloway M, Szyldowski G, et al. Intraoperative brachytherapy following thoracoscopic wedge resection of stage I lung cancer. Chest 1998;114(4):1112–5.

[28] Santos R, Colonias A, Parda D, et al. Comparison between sublobar resection and 125 iodine brachytherapy after sublobar resection in high-risk patients with stage I non-small-cell lung cancer. Surgery 2003;134:691–7.

[29] Fernando HC, Santos RS, Benfield JR, et al. Lobar and sublobar resection with and without brachytherapy for small stage IA NSCLC. J Thorac Cardiovasc Surg 2005;129(2):261–7.

[30] Birdas TJ, Koehler RP, Colonias A, et al. Sublobar resection with brachytherapy versus lobectomy for stage Ib non-small cell lung cancer. Ann Thorac Surg 2006;81(2):434–8.

[31] Patel AN, Santos RS, DeHoyos A, et al. Clinical trials of peripheral stage I (T1N0M0) non-small cell lung cancer. Semin Thorac Cardiovasc Surg 2003;15:421–30.

[32] Jones DR, Stiles BM, Denlinger CE, et al. Pulmonary segmentectomy: results and complications. Ann Thorac Surg 2003;76(2):343–8 [discussion: 348–9].

[33] Schuchert MJ, Pettiford BL, Keeley S, et al. Efficacy of anatomic segmentectomy and the importance of surgical margin: tumor diameter ratio in the treatment of stage I non-small cell lung cancer (NSCLC). Abstract presented orally at the 43 Annual Meeting of the Society of Thoracic Surgeons. San Diego (CA), January 29–31, 2007.

[34] Fisher B, Anderson S, Bryant J, et al. Twenty-year follow-up of a randomized trial comparing total mastectomy, lumpectomy, and lumpectomy plus irradiation for the treatment of invasive breast cancer. N Engl J Med 2002;347(16):1233–41.

[35] Erret LE, Wilson J, Chiu RC-J, et al. Wedge resection as an alternative procedure for peripheral bronchogenic carcinomas in poor-risk patients. J Thorac Cardiovasc Surg 1985;90:656–61.

[36] Ikeda N, Hayashi A, Miura Y, et al. Present strategy of lung cancer screening and surgical management. Ann Thorac Cardiovasc Surg 2005;11(6):363–6.

[37] Henschke CI. I-ELCAP Investigators. CT screening for lung cancer: update 2005. Surg Oncol Clin N Am 2005;14(4):761–76.

[38] Uematsu M. Stereotactic radiation therapy for non-small cell lung cancer. Nippon Geka Gakkai Zasshi 2002;103(2):256–7.

[39] Fernando HC, de Hoyos A, Landreneau RJ, et al. Radiofrequency ablation for the treatment of non-small cell lung cancer in marginal surgical

candidates. J Thorac Cardiovasc Surg 2005;129(3): 639–44.

[40] El-Sherif A, Luketich JD, Landreneau RJ, et al. New therapeutic approaches for early-stage non-small cell lung cancer. J Surg Oncol 2005;14(1): 27–32.

[41] Nagata Y, Takayama K, Matsuo Y, et al. Clinical outcomes of a phase I/II study of 48 Gy of stereotactic body radiotherapy in 4 fractions for primary lung cancer using a stereotactic body frame. Int J Radiat Oncol Biol Phys 2005;63(5):1427–31.

[42] Inoue M, Minami M, Shiono H, et al. Clinicopathologic study of resected, peripheral, small-sized, non-small cell lung cancer tumors of 2 cm or less in diameter: pleural invasion and increase of serum carcinoembryonic antigen level as predictors of nodal involvement. J Thorac Cardiovasc Surg 2006; 131(5):988–93.

[43] Noirclerc M. Muscle-sparing thoracotomy. Ann Thorac Surg 1989;47(2):330b.

[44] Swerc MF, Landreneau RJ, Santos RS, et al. Mini-thoracotomy combined with mechanically stapled bronchial and vascular ligation for anatomical lung resection. Ann Thorac Surg 2004;77(6):1904–9.

[45] Miller JI Jr, Landreneau RJ, Wright CE, et al. A comparative study of buttressed versus nonbuttressed staple line in pulmonary resections. Ann Thorac Surg 2001;71(1):319–22.

[46] Gagarine A, Urschel JD, Miller JD, et al. Effect of fibrin glue on air leak and length of hospital stay after pulmonary lobectomy. J Cardiovasc Surg (Torino) 2003;44(6):771–3.

[47] Lee W, Daly BD, DiPetrillo TA, et al. Limited resection for non-small cell lung cancer: observed local control with implantation of I-125 brachytherapy seeds. Ann Thorac Surg 2003;75(1):237–42.

[48] Shiraishi T, Shirakusa T, Iwasaki A, et al. Video-assisted thoracoscopic surgery (VATS) segmentectomy for small peripheral lung cancer tumors. Surg Endosc 2004;18:1657–62.

ELSEVIER
SAUNDERS

Thorac Surg Clin 17 (2007) 191–201

THORACIC
SURGERY
CLINICS

Management of the Peripheral Small Ground-Glass Opacities

Junji Yoshida, MD, PhD

Division of Thoracic Surgery, Department of Thoracic Oncology,
National Cancer Center Hospital East, 6-5-1, Kashiwanoha, Kashiwa, Chiba, 277-8577, Japan

The introduction of new equipment and techniques normally brings new discoveries. So it was with the introduction of CT. The first CT scans were very slow and had poor resolution in general, but if great care was taken, small areas could have high-resolution CT (HRCT), also known as a "thin-section CT scan." The initial investigations were for diffuse parenchymal changes like fibrosis and interstitial changes. Radiologists soon noticed, however, well-defined areas that had a "ground-glass" quality. The parenchyma in these areas was not solid like a normal carcinoma, but neither were they like normal lung parenchyma.

In the early 1990s, radiologists and CT scanner manufacturers cooperated to develop low-dose spiral scanning CT machines. CT scanning was much faster, the resolution much better, and patient radiation exposure was much lower. HRCT also became much easier to perform, with better resolution. Many more CT scans were performed. With the increased number of CT scans, the number of ground-glass opacity (GGO) lesions found increased. Surgeons removed them and discovered that, even though they were not solid, they were often carcinomas: they were bronchioloalveolar carcinomas (BAC).

They seemed to have some different characteristics and natural history, however, than solid carcinomas. Generally, they were small; most were slow growing. Additionally, some patients had more than one GGO, and the multiple GGOs were in different lobes. This presented some

challenges to surgeons. The more lung parenchyma removed the more impact on lung function and patient quality of life.

Lung cancer surgical treatment has been a progression of less and less parenchymal removal and less impact on lung function. The first lung cancer treatment was pneumonectomy [1]. It took almost 20 years before it was replaced by lobectomy [2]. Limited resection has not been widely accepted or used. It has been tried, however, in patients unfit for lobectomy, resulted in satisfactory outcomes, and has been widely accepted as a compromise [3].

In 1995, the Lung Cancer Study Group, after performing the only prospective randomized trial on limited resection versus lobectomy for stage IA patients, concluded lobectomy was the appropriate surgical treatment and limited resection was not, because limited resection resulted in worse outcomes [4]. Even though they were small stage IA tumors, they were still invasive. As a result, thoracic surgeons were cautious and very selective in performing limited resection on lung cancer patients. It was used mostly where the patient had reduced lung function, even before surgery. Limited resection could be used routinely, or even encouraged, if a tumor was known to be noninvasive or minimally invasive. The problem was finding or identifying noninvasive or minimally invasive tumors. It was reported that even in peripheral lung cancers smaller than 1 cm in diameter, an invasive nature was observed in almost half of the tumors [5]. It was evident tumor size alone is not a useful positive indicator for limited resection.

A GGO is defined as an area of hazy increased attenuation of the lung, but with preservation of

This work is supported in part by a Grant-in-Aid for Cancer Research from the Ministry of Health, Labour and Welfare, Japan.

E-mail address: jyoshida@east.ncc.go.jp

thoracic.theclinics.com

bronchial and vascular margins [6]. They are often invisible on a conventional plain chest radiograph. With the clinical introduction of HRCT in the mid-1980s, researchers used it in evaluating diffuse peripheral lung diseases described as GGOs [7]. Kuriyama and colleagues [8] found that most of the well-differentiated or moderately differentiated papillary adenocarcinoma showing a peripheral fluffy zone on HRCT correlated well with tumor cells lining the alveolar walls observed in pathologic studies.

The introduction of low-dose spiral CT made HRCT scanning easier and less time-consuming. In the early 1990s, with more GGOs being found, attention was still directed mostly at diffuse diseases with a ground-glass appearance [9,10]. But Koizumi and colleagues [11] found cloudy, or GGO, nodules clearly demarcated on HRCT were mostly well-differentiated adenocarcinoma, mainly bronchioloalveolar type with little or no central scar. Engeler and colleagues [12] described the pathologic basis of GGOs as any condition that decreases the lung parenchyma air fraction without totally obliterating the alveoli.

In 1995, Noguchi and colleagues [13] developed a six-class system for small adenocarcinoma (Table 1). They concluded Noguchi's type A, a localized BAC, and type B, a localized BAC with foci of collapse, should be considered in situ peripheral adenocarcinoma. Those with stromal

destruction, with foci of active fibroblastic proliferation, were Noguchi type C and were an advanced stage of types A and B. Although the conclusions were speculative at the time, Japanese researchers were encouraged that there was evidence that type A and B tumors are in situ carcinomas. If they were truly in situ carcinomas, limited resection would be the management of choice for Noguchi types A and B.

Low-dose spiral CT technology provides an improved lung cancer CT screening method. Extensive use began both in Japan [14,15] and in New York [16]. Screening researchers found localized or focal GGO lesions (Fig. 1). Even with considerable presurgery CT section examination, not knowing what they were, surgeons did standard resections and found many were localized BACs. Pathologic examination found some were not carcinomas, however, but atypical adenomatous hyperplasia (AAH), and others were inflammatory changes. Kuriyama and colleagues [17] reported that GGO or subsolid nodules identified on HRCT corresponded to the lepidic growth pattern of localized BAC. As these nodules grow, the lepidic framework of the lung stroma is disrupted, indicating stromal invasion [18] and resulting in pleural indentation and convergence of the bronchovascular structures [19].

The reports by Koizumi, Kuriyama, Noguchi and others provided researchers at the National

Table 1
Noguchi's classification of small adenocarcinoma of the lung

Type	Description
A	LBAC
B	LBAC with foci of collapse of alveolar structure
C	LBAC with foci of active fibroblastic proliferation
D	Poorly differentiated adenocarcinoma
E	Tubular adenocarcinoma
F	Papillary adenocarcinoma with compressive and destructive growth

Abbreviation: LBAC, localized bronchioloalveolar carcinoma.

Data from Noguchi M, Morikawa A, Kawasaki M, et al. Small adenocarcinoma of the lung: histologic characteristics and prognosis. Cancer 1995;75:2844–52.

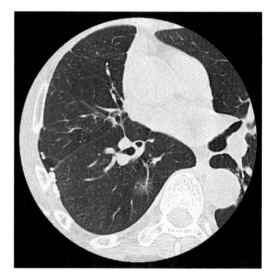

Fig. 1. Typical localized GGO lesion. This lesion proved to be a Noguchi type B tumor.

Cancer Center Hospital East with a conceptual model for GGO initiation, development, and progression. Based on the model, trials were developed to validate the model and learn more about GGOs. It seemed GGO lung tumors on HRCT were likely noninvasive or minimally invasive cancers, which could be curatively resected using just limited resection rather than lobectomy and lymph node dissection. This would reduce the lung function impact. The reduction would be even less if there were GGOs in more than one lobe.

Based on this thinking, two GGO treatment trials were initiated by wedge resection or segmentectomy rather than lobectomy. One trial is complete with very good conclusive results. The other trial is still in process, but with good initial indications. No patient in either trial has had a recurrence or died of lung cancer.

Intraoperative Noguchi subtype diagnosis trial

Objectives and methods

In 1998, a prospective clinical trial was started of limited resection for probable in situ adenocarcinoma in the lung periphery [20]. The objective was to confirm limited resection efficacy in patients with Noguchi type A and B tumors. Noguchi's classification was determined intraoperatively by frozen section examination.

Patients with a tumor smaller than 2 cm in diameter diagnosed or suspected as a clinical T1N0M0 carcinoma in the lung periphery based on a CT scan were enrolled. They had to have a GGO on HRCT and the tumor had to lack pleural indentations or vascular convergence. Patients with a malignancy history within the past 5 years and those unfit for lobectomy and systematic lymph node dissection were excluded.

Fig. 2 shows the treatment flow chart. Wedge or segmental resection was performed, depending on the tumor location. Three-port procedures were performed when the tumor was on the lung "outer surface," or when the tumor was shallow or hard enough to palpate directly with one or two fingers through the ports. When it was impossible to determine the tumor location or its margin through the ports, the procedure was converted to a small 5-cm thoracotomy. When a tumor was deep in the middle of a segment, segmentectomy was chosen. Also, when a tumor could not be localized during surgery, a segmentectomy was performed to avoid missing the tumor.

The pathologist immediately, by frozen section, examined the specimen. If the tumor was confirmed Noguchi type A or B, and the resection margin was larger than 1 cm, the patient was closed up and followed on an outpatient basis. If the margin was not sufficient, additional margin was resected. If the tumor was a primary malignancy, but not a Noguchi type A or B, lobectomy and systematic lymph node dissection were performed.

It is fairly difficult to perform Noguchi classification on an uninflated, typically stained frozen section [21]. To facilitate the examination, several additional methods were used in the trial. With no obvious specimen bronchus or

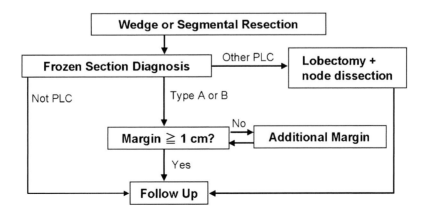

Fig. 2. Treatment sequence. PLC, primary lung cancer. (*From* Yoshida J, Nagai K, Yokose T, et al. Limited resection trial for pulmonary ground-glass opacity nodules: fifty-case experience. J Thorac Cardiovasc Surg 2005;129:992; with permission.)

bronchiole in a wedge resection specimen for phosphate-buffered saline injection, specimen inflation to facilitate alveolar structure examination is difficult. To inflate the resected specimen's alveolar structure with phosphate-buffered saline, the pathologist used a technique known, but not normally used, in neoplastic lung disease diagnosis [22]. With the specimen in a closed, phosphate-buffered saline-filled syringe, the piston was repeatedly pulled back. The alveolar air bubbles out, is replaced with phosphate-buffered saline, and the specimen becomes heavier and sinks (Fig. 3).

After slicing the specimen into 2-mm thick slices and a second reinflation, the pathologist stereoscopically examined the slices looking for the most severe signs of alveolar structure destruction. The maximum stromal destruction slices or the largest tumor dimension slice were frozen and cut by cryostat, stained, and examined microscopically.

In addition to routine hematoxylin-eosin staining, the pathologist correctly thought Victoria-blue van Gieson's staining would improve Noguchi's classification accuracy, clearly identifying lung stroma elastic fiber destruction. Victoria-blue van Gieson's staining reveals whether or not the alveolar wall elastic fibers are intact, providing a powerful aid in identifying stromal destruction [23]. If the elastic fibers were destroyed by tumor cells, the tumor was diagnosed as Noguchi type C, whereas if intact, the classification was type A or B.

Patients are followed-up on an outpatient basis at least every 6 months by physical check-up, plain chest radiograph, and laboratory tests. Patients who underwent limited resection for Noguchi type A or B disease have chest CT every year.

Results and comments

This prospective protocol study started in August 1998, and the fiftieth and last patient was enrolled in October 2002. GGOs are a small subset of the general lung cancer population. This was only 5.3% of all the resected lung cancer patients during the same period. There were 20 men and 30 women, with ages ranging from 30 to 77 years (average, 61 years). Tumor sizes ranged from 2 to 21 mm (average, 11 mm). Thirty patients had wedge resection, 6 segmentectomy, and 14 lobectomy with lymph node dissection. Nineteen of the 30 wedge procedures were performed thoracoscopically by three-port access, and the other 11 needed a small thoracotomy. Segmentectomy and lobectomy were done through a muscle-sparing typically 12-cm thoracotomy. Initially, because little was known of GGOs, it was unclear whether these lesions could be localized and palpated. It was found, however, that the GGO-containing lung parenchyma had a different texture than the surrounding normal parenchyma.

Although it was estimated routinely to take 15 to 20 minutes, during the trial Noguchi classification assessment took about an hour because of the extensive image recording required for trial study purposes. There were 2 type A tumors, 23 type B tumors, 15 type C tumors, 5 AAHs, 4 fibroses, and 1 granuloma. One initial frozen section type B diagnosis was revised to type C after postoperative pathologic study. After detailed discussion, the patient chose not to have any further treatment. He is still alive without any signs of recurrence after more than 7.5 years. His protocol was modified, with a bi-annual CT examination performed for the first 3 years.

The other 14 Noguchi type C tumor patients, whose diagnoses were confirmed by postoperative

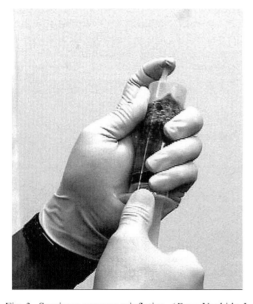

Fig. 3. Specimen vacuum reinflation. (*From* Yoshida J, Nagai K, Yokose T, et al. Limited resection trial for pulmonary ground-glass opacity nodules: fifty-case experience. J Thorac Cardiovasc Surg 2005;129:993; with permission.)

pathologic study, underwent lobectomy and systematic lymph node dissection following the frozen section diagnosis. Detailed pathologic study after surgery found no nodal involvement, pulmonary metastases, lymphatic permeation, or vascular invasion in all type Noguchi C specimens. Even though they were more invasive than type A or B tumors, they were fairly localized diseases and demonstrated little invasiveness.

There was no correlation between tumor size and subtype (Table 2). All Noguchi type C tumors were 1 cm or greater, however, whereas other subtypes included subcentimeter tumors. This strengthens the suggestion that limited resection is strongly indicated when a GGO tumor is less than 1 cm. This contradicts a previous review [5] and Mayo Clinic's reported data on subcentimeter lung cancers [24]. This is probably caused by those series including non-GGO or solid lesions.

No morbidity or mortality has occurred. During the follow-up period, with a range of 49 to 98 months (median, 80 months), as this article was being written (November 2006), there have been no recurrences. Follow-up contact was with one type B patient 3 years after resection. Considering the slow-growing nature of GGO lesions [25–27], less than 7 years of median follow-up period is not long enough to conclude the disease cured. Follow-up has to be continued for an additional 3 to 4 years. The current results, however, are convincing, Noguchi's criteria seem useful, and the conclusions valid.

Table 2
Histologic subtype and tumor size distribution in resected specimens

Subtype	No. of cases	Range (mm)	Median (mm)	Resection type (W/S/L)
Type A	2	9–10	—	1/1/0
Type B	23	6–21	12	21/2/0
Type C	15	10–19	14	1/0/14
Atypical adenomatous hyperplasia	5	5–14	8	2/3/0
Fibrosis	4	6–15	10	4/0/0
Granuloma	1	6	—	1/0/0

Abbreviation: W/S/L, wedge resection/segmentectomy/lobectomy plus lymph node dissection, in numbers of patients.
Data from Yoshida J, Nagai K, Yokose T, et al. Limited resection trial for pulmonary ground-glass opacity nodules: fifty-case experience. J Thorac Cardiovasc Surg 2005;129:991–6.

The first trial showed Noguchi's classification by intraoperative frozen section can be very accurate. With a median follow-up period of over 6.5 years there have been no recurrences. At this time, it is convincing that limited resection is sufficient for Noguchi type A and B tumors less than 20 mm.

Detailed postoperative pathologic study of the Noguchi type C tumors found no nodal involvement, pulmonary metastases, lymphatic permeation, or vascular invasion. This suggests all eligible GGO lung cancers in the study, including the type C tumors, might have been radically managed with only limited resection. One type C tumor had only limited resection. The patient decided to not have further treatment, and he is still alive with no recurrence.

High-resolution CT and lavage trial

The basis

A common question is, "Isn't frozen section Noguchi's classification too demanding or time consuming?" Perhaps, and it also requires a highly experienced pathologist. Additionally, the surgeons and operating room staff were very patient while the trial level pathologic examination took place.

Because all the GGO lung cancers in the previous trial might have been radically managed with only limited resection, with its lower lung function impact, was there a way to simplify the procedure? The search began to find better ways to select suitable patients, and establish a clean, noncancerous resected margin. Several articles by Japanese researchers showed good correlation between radiologic and pathologic findings in early lung adenocarcinoma [17,19,28–30]. This, along with an earlier investigation [31,32], gave a hint on how to find suitable candidates. For negative margin confirmation, an interesting technique using lavage and cytologic examination was found, first reported by Higashiyama and colleagues [33].

As a leading edge trial, there were no established means or criteria for radiologic identification of noninvasive, in situ lung cancer. It might be the ultimate goal of CT or MRI microscopy, but it does not exist today at the patient level. HRCT findings are fairly suggestive of pathologically minimally invasive GGO lung cancer, however, and they are available today. The decision was made to start the current trial using existing information and techniques.

Objectives and methods

The current trial's objectives are to confirm limited resection efficacy in patients with HRCT-indicated minimally invasive lung cancer, and to confirm intraoperative cytology as a negative margin indicator and reliable margin nonrecurrence predictor. Enrollment requires patients with a tumor smaller than 2 cm in maximum dimension, diagnosed or suspected as a clinical T1N0M0 carcinoma in the lung periphery based on a CT scan. They had to have a HRCT scan indicating a pure or mixed GGO nodule with a tumor disappearance ratio (TDR) 0.5 or greater.

TDR is defined as follows (Fig. 4). On a HRCT slice, the maximum tumor diameter is measured on lung setting (DL). On mediastinal setting, the ground-glass area disappears leaving only the consolidation area. The remaining consolidation area maximum diameter is measured (DM). TDR is calculated as 1 – DM/DL. Fig. 5 shows an example of TDR measurement and calculation. A ground-glass diameter of 17 mm and consolidation diameter of 6 mm yields a 0.65 TDR. The tumor proved to be a Noguchi type B. Based on length measurement, the solid region is confirmed as a maximum 25% of the total slice displayed GGO tumor area. The solid area is a relatively small fraction of the total tumor area. Thinking in terms of volume, eligible patients have a rather small solid volume, which is less than 12.5% if the tumor is a sphere.

Patients with a malignancy history within 5 years, and those unfit for lobectomy and systematic lymph node dissection, are excluded. The end point is 5-year local recurrence-free survival. With a trial size of 100 patients, the quit-the-trial rule is

if there are two or more local recurrence cases among the initial 30 cases or three or more among the initial 60.

Fig. 6 shows the treatment flow chart. A wedge or segmental resection is performed using the same criteria as the first trial. Using the method described next, the cytologist examines the specimen margin immediately. If the cytology result is cancer positive, additional margin is resected and cytologic examination repeated. If the second cytologic examination is also positive, a routine lobectomy and systematic lymph node dissection are performed.

To establish a clean margin faster and easier, the method described by Higashiyama and colleagues [33] is used. The used stapling cartridges are washed repeatedly with 50 mL of saline. Endo GIA Universal Roticulator cartridges (USSC, Norwalk, Connecticut) are usually used, which are very easy to wash. Both the knife in the shaft and the anvil faces are flushed using a washing syringe from the shaft end (Fig. 7). The washing saline is centrifuged. The sediment is Papanicolaou stained and examined for cancer cells. This procedure does not take long, and is less skill sensitive than pathologic examination.

Patients are followed-up on an outpatient basis every 6 months by chest CT for the first 3 years, and annually thereafter. This is more frequent than the first trial because of the greater uncertainty. Even though the trial end point is 5 years, it is not known for sure how long after that. Like the first study, follow-up is expected to last at least 5 years and maybe 10 years.

The primary end point is the 5-year local recurrence-free survival. Also, intraoperative cytology as a negative margin indicator and reliable margin nonrecurrence predictor will be evaluated. It is believed that secondary benefits will be less lung function impact, and if necessary, a surgical second chance. The first trial's patients have had those same benefits and opportunities. This study protocol was reviewed by the National Cancer Center Hospital East Institutional Review Board and was approved in October 2003.

Results

This prospective study started in November 2003, and 29 patients have been enrolled as of October 2006. Like the first study, it is a rather small fraction of all patients treated over this period, only 3.7%. There were 9 men and 20 women. Tumor sizes ranged from 7 to 20 mm on

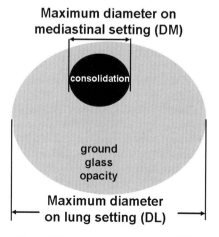

Maximum diameter on mediastinal setting (DM)

consolidation

ground glass opacity

Maximum diameter on lung setting (DL)

Fig. 4. Schematic measurement for TDR.

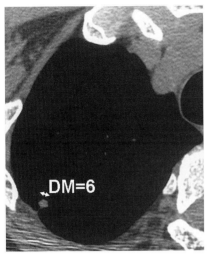
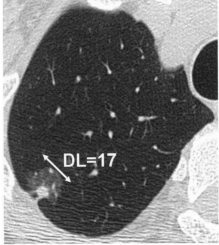

Fig. 5. TDR calculation example. DL, maximum tumor diameter on lung setting; DM, consolidation area maximum diameter on mediastinal setting.

HRCT, with a 15 mm average. Twenty-eight patients had a wedge resection, and one a segmentectomy. All the cases were started thoracoscopically. If the tumor could not be located confidently, even with an Endo-finger through a 2-cm video-assisted thorascopic surgery port incision, there was no hesitation to enlarge the best located 2-cm incision to 5 cm. If there was uncertainty about lesion location even with a 5-cm incision, a 10-cm incision was chosen, which allowed segmentectomy if necessary. Two of the patients needed the muscle-sparing 10-cm standard thoracotomy.

There were 5 type A tumors, 13 type B tumors, 7 type C tumors, and 1 unclassifiable adenocarcinoma. There were three overtreated or overexamined patients with inflammatory changes. It was suspected that two of the three patients had inflammatory changes and we recommended

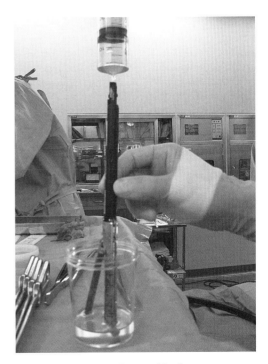

Fig. 7. Stapling cartridge lavage.

Fig. 6. Current trial treatment sequence. CME, cytologic margin evaluation.

a watchful waiting strategy. They wanted immediate resection, however, for emotional reasons. None of the cancers, including the type C, had vessel invasion. There seems to be a trend toward lower TDR in type C tumors compared with type As, but the differences between the Noguchi's subtypes were not significant (Fig. 8). As expected in a 3-year old trial, there have been no recurrences, but it is far too early and the results far too preliminary to conclude anything.

Other trials

The first prospective limited resection trial for GGO lung cancer patients was reported by Yamato and colleagues [34]. Based on a protocol similar to the first trial, they enrolled 42 patients in almost 4 years, and limited resection was completed in 36 patients (wedge resection in 34 and segmentectomy in 2). Although the median follow-up period was short at 30 months, all patients were alive without signs of recurrence.

Watanabe and colleagues [35] reported in 2002 on limited resection results in 20 patients with pure GGO lesions accumulated over 5 years. The study design did not report whether or not it was prospective. They had a standard practice for pure GGO patients. Twenty patients elected the surgery and underwent limited resection. Of these, 17 patients had noninvasive BAC (wedge resection in 14 and segmentectomy in 3) and 3 AAH. Although they performed intraoperative frozen section examination, the results did not alter their surgical procedures. The median follow-up

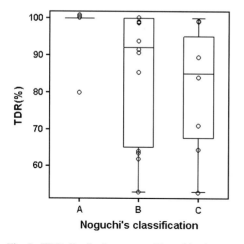

Fig. 8. TDR distribution among Noguchi subtypes.

time was also short at 32 months, but there were no cancer deaths or recurrences.

Yamada and Kohno [36] reported on a prospective trial for pure GGO patients in 2004, with a protocol similar to the National Cancer Center Hospital East first trial. They included multiple GGO patients, on whom segmentectomy or lobectomy was performed. Thirty-nine patients were enrolled in 25 months, and 30 had solitary GGO lesions. Of the 30 solitary lesion patients, eight had AAH; 20 localized BAC (Noguchi type A or B); and two type C tumors. The nine other patients were multilesion patients. Their lesions totaled 8 AAHs and 24 Noguchi type A or B. The mean follow-up period for patients with localized BAC was 29 months, and all patients remained alive and no recurrence of disease was observed.

With the small numbers of patients presenting with GGOs, all of these, including the author's, are single-arm, limited resection-only studies. Patient numbers are small, patients are not randomized, and follow-up periods are short in a situation where patients may be at risk for recurrence for up to 10 years or maybe even longer. With the excellent survival compared with normal lung cancer patient survival even at the short interval, however, the current results are convincing and the concept of some GGOs being noninvasive or minimally invasive lung cancer seems valid.

National Cancer Center Hospital East ground-glass opacity management strategy

These trials, a good pathologist, and the treatment team have improved and demonstrated the usefulness of the GGO development model. It seems that BAC develops, and rather than developing as a solid mass from the start, spreads along the alveolar walls. This wall thickening is what causes the radiologic haziness. Identifying the edge where the spread stops can present challenges. Sometimes it appears to be a clear break, whereas other times it appears to be a bit fuzzy. It is uncertain whether this is caused by histopathologic factors, CT processing, or display settings, but it requires careful examination. During this initial wall-following period, the tumor is growing rather noninvasively. Generally, the tumor size is increasing but at a slow rate.

At some point the carcinoma changes and invasive aspects develop. The growth rate along the alveolar walls can increase. The carcinoma cells can also start breaking through the alveolar walls and spread into the surrounding stroma. The GGO begins to develop consolidated solid areas. In these solid areas, the alveolar structure is destroyed and the alveolar air space collapses, pulling in the surrounding parenchyma, resulting in pleural indentation and vascular convergence. Because of the collapse, nodule volume reduction can occur and the lesion maximum dimensions can actually shrink rather than grow. Use of TDR addresses this issue, because the TDR decreases along with the shrinking total maximum tumor dimension or volume. With the appearance of solid areas, there is a greater chance of venous or lymphatic involvement. Appearance of any of these is a strong invasiveness indicator and reason to soon schedule a surgical biopsy.

These surgical intervention trials have shown GGO lung cancers are mostly localized BAC, and are noninvasive or minimally invasive [20,34–36]. Invasiveness or stromal destruction is reasonably predictable based on HRCT findings [17–19,28–32]. If a mixed GGO has a relatively large consolidation area, the lesion should strongly be suspected as an invasive BAC, and immediate physical biopsy is recommended. If lung cancer is confirmed, standard lobectomy and systematic node dissection is recommended. If an experienced, skilled pathologist is available, however, lobectomy may not be required. By using intraoperative frozen section, invasiveness and stromal destruction of the specimen can be determined, and the Noguchi type determined. For Noguchi type A or B tumors, and probably type C tumors with a minimal fibroblastic focus, limited resection is a reasonable treatment choice.

If the HRCT shows a pure GGO or mixed GGO with a small consolidation area, the tumor is most likely a localized BAC with no or minimal stromal destruction. Observational studies have shown they are slow-growing and often remain unchanged for several years [25–27]. For these GGO lesions, there is no need for immediate resection.

Because some GGO lesions, and in particular pure GGO or mixed GGOs with minimal consolidation area, are only inflammatory changes, observation with antibiotics for several weeks is recommended. This is particularly the case if pleural indentation or vascular convergence is not found. Fuzzy, or indistinct GGO margin appearance often is an indicator of an inflammatory condition. The more defined, the greater the need for surgical intervention. If the GGO disappears on a follow-up CT, the inflammatory nature is confirmed. This is the strategy leading CT screening programs recommend [27,37].

Even if a high TDR GGO lesion does not disappear after a course of antibiotics and a repeat CT scan, because of GGO's slow-growing nature, immediate surgical resection is still not recommended. Follow-up CT on a 3- or even 6-month interval to monitor growth and edge condition is appropriate. If a lesion remains unchanged after a year's monitoring, changing to an annual follow-up CT seems adequate. When the tumor shows sufficient growth, exceeding 10 to 15 mm in diameter, its consolidation area grows, or the margin becomes well defined, it is time for resection.

There can be a concern as to what is an appropriate "small" consolidation area. The author currently uses a TDR of 0.5 or greater. This seems valid, but needs to be monitored for continued validity. Additionally, two-dimensional tools are mainly being used; three-dimensional tool use might provide additional insight.

Summary and future directions

There are two strongly confounding issues concerning GGO trials to date. One is that GGOs are slow growing, and need long follow-up monitoring periods, estimated now to be 10 years. Two, only small numbers of patients with GGO present at any one institution, and so it takes time to accumulate a trial population, extending the time until unquestionable results are available. Meanwhile, results to date indicate that these are noninvasive or minimally invasive tumors and early limited resection seems to be very successful. There seems to be reason to report results as quickly as possible for use by others. These two issues are confounding factors. For the patients, however, early data may well be useful.

Because of the often-described slow-growing nature of GGO cancers, it is too early at this time to recommend a fixed management strategy for these lesions. More follow-up data are needed at a median follow-up period of 10 years or so.

These trials, however, have improved the GGO development conceptual model. The tumor pathology studies confirmed what was expected to be found based on HRCT. More GGO development attributes were identified that can be used for GGO treatment staging. Based on the GGO stage, the patient may not have to undergo immediate surgery. From the current trial data, the surgery may not have to be lobectomy, but limited resection with reduced lung function impact.

Many studies have shown a mixed GGO with a large consolidation area (low TDR) needs quick intervention. A pure GGO or a mixed GGO with a small consolidation area (high TDR) can be observed, however, with a short-term antibiotics course. Even if it does not go away after antibiotics, watchful waiting with a biannual or annual follow-up CT is acceptable until it grows over 10 to 15 mm, its consolidation area grows, the margin becomes better defined, or pleural indentation or vascular convergence occurs. The key here is growth. Either overall lesion growth of greater than 10 to 15 mm, appearance of, or increasing consolidation area with pleural indentation or vascular convergence is growth.

When it is time for resection, limited resection based on intraoperative Noguchi classification by frozen section is accurate and a reasonable alternative to classic lobectomy. So far, patient selection based solely on HRCT findings seems valid. HRCT enables one to know with high reliability if noninvasive or minimally invasive lung cancers will be found before surgery begins. However, there is a need for more experience by others with the diagnostic criteria.

The number of GGO nodules is small, only about 4% of all resected lung cancer patients so far. Even fewer may be seen on repeat screening after the initial screening. In the author's earlier trial, it took 4 years to accumulate 50 patients, and 7 years to have results. There is a 100-patient goal for the current single-institution HRCT-based trial, but in 3 years, there are only 29 patients. There are thoughts of ending the current trial at a 50-case accumulation. Although it is not the initial goal, it will provide sufficient confidence in treating GGO cancers as localized disease.

Experience to date indicates that pure GGOs or high-TDR GGOs are lung cancers that have not yet become invasive. For these not yet invasive tumors, limited resection seems to be an appropriate treatment, even without double-arm studies. The survival rates are significantly better than historical survival rates for invasive lung cancers.

Because HRCT seems to predict noninvasive or minimally invasive GGO lung cancers with high reliability, less invasive treatments have greater appeal. Radiofrequency ablation, cryosurgery, stereotactic radiation therapy, or particle beam radiation therapy might be used as a radical and less invasive treatment. They might appeal to patients who elect to wait rather than have immediate surgery. These modalities need to be examined in future trials, selecting patients based on HRCT findings. Even at this stage, however, it seems that a lower-impact surgery (wedge resection or segmentectomy) is curative for this noninvasive or minimally invasive subset of lung cancers.

Acknowledgment

The author thanks Brian Curry, communication consultant, Chester Springs, Pennsylvania, for his continuous help in focusing on clearness, conciseness, and clarity.

References

[1] Graham EA, Singer JJ. Landmark article Oct 28, 1933. Successful removal of an entire lung for carcinoma of the bronchus. By Evarts A. Graham and J. J. Singer. JAMA 1984;251(2):257–60.

[2] Churchill ED, Sweet RH, Shutter L, et al. The surgical management of carcinoma of the lung: a study of cases treated at the Massachusetts General Hospital from 1930–1950. J Thorac Cardiovasc Surg 1950;20: 349–65.

[3] Miller JI Jr. Limited resection of bronchogenic carcinoma in the patient with impaired pulmonary function. Ann Thorac Surg 1993;56(3):769–71.

[4] Ginsberg RJ, Rubinstein LV. Randomized trial of lobectomy versus limited resection for T1 N0 non-small cell lung cancer. Lung Cancer Study Group. Ann Thorac Surg 1995;60(3):615–22.

[5] Yoshida J, Nagai K, Yokose T, et al. Primary peripheral lung carcinoma smaller than 1 cm in diameter. Chest 1998;114(3):710–2.

[6] Austin JH, Muller NL, Friedman PJ, et al. Glossary of terms for CT of the lungs: recommendations of the Nomenclature Committee of the Fleischner Society. Radiology 1996;200(2):327–31.

[7] Nakata H, Kimoto T, Nakayama T, et al. Diffuse peripheral lung disease: evaluation by high-resolution computed tomography. Radiology 1985; 157(1):181–5.

[8] Kuriyama K, Tateishi R, Doi O, et al. CT-pathologic correlation in small peripheral lung cancers. AJR Am J Roentgenol 1987;149(6):1139–43.

[9] Zwirewich CV, Mayo JR, Muller NL. Low-dose high-resolution CT of lung parenchyma. Radiology 1991;180(2):413–7.

[10] Vock P, Soucek M. Spiral computed tomography in the assessment of focal and diffuse lung disease. J Thorac Imaging 1993;8(4):283–90.

[11] Koizumi N, Akita S, Sakai K, et al. Cloudy nodule on HRCT: a new clinico-radiologic entity of pulmonary adenocarcinoma. Radiat Med 1995;13(6): 273–8.

[12] Engeler CE, Tashjian JH, Trenkner SW, et al. Ground-glass opacity of the lung parenchyma: a guide to analysis with high-resolution CT. AJR Am J Roentgenol 1993;160(2):249–51.

[13] Noguchi M, Morikawa A, Kawasaki M, et al. Small adenocarcinoma of the lung: histologic characteristics and prognosis. Cancer 1995;75(12):2844–52.

[14] Kaneko M, Eguchi K, Ohmatsu H, et al. Peripheral lung cancer: screening and detection with low-dose spiral CT versus radiography. Radiology 1996; 201(3):798–802.

[15] Sone S, Takashima S, Li F, et al. Mass screening for lung cancer with mobile spiral computed tomography scanner. Lancet 1998;351(9111):1242–5.

[16] Henschke CI, McCauley DI, Yankelevitz DF, et al. Early Lung Cancer Action Project: overall design and findings from baseline screening. Lancet 1999; 354(9173):99–105.

[17] Kuriyama K, Seto M, Kasugai T, et al. Ground-glass opacity on thin-section CT: value in differentiating subtypes of adenocarcinoma of the lung. AJR Am J Roentgenol 1999;173(2):465–9.

[18] Eto T, Suzuki H, Honda A, et al. The changes of the stromal elastotic framework in the growth of peripheral lung adenocarcinomas. Cancer 1996;77(4): 646–56.

[19] Yang Z, Sone S, Takashima S, et al. Small peripheral carcinomas of the lung: thin-section CT and pathologic correlation. Eur Radiol 1999;9(9):1819–25.

[20] Yoshida J, Nagai K, Yokose T, et al. Limited resection trial for pulmonary ground-glass opacity nodules: fifty-case experience. J Thorac Cardiovasc Surg 2005;129(5):991–6.

[21] Mori M, Chiba R, Takahashi T. Atypical adenomatous hyperplasia of the lung and its differentiation from adenocarcinoma: characterization of atypical cells by morphometry and multivariate cluster analysis. Cancer 1993;72(8):2331–40.

[22] van Kuppevelt TH, Robbesom AA, Versteeg EM, et al. Restoration by vacuum inflation of original alveolar dimensions in small human lung specimens. Eur Respir J 2000;15(4):771–7.

[23] Goto K, Yokose T, Kodama T, et al. Detection of early invasion on the basis of basement membrane destruction in small adenocarcinomas of the lung and its clinical implications. Mod Pathol 2001; 14(12):1237–45.

[24] Miller DL, Rowland CM, Deschamps C, et al. Surgical treatment of non-small cell lung cancer 1 cm or less in diameter. Ann Thorac Surg 2002;73(5): 1545–50.

[25] Hasegawa M, Sone S, Takashima S, et al. Growth rate of small lung cancers detected on mass CT screening. Br J Radiol 2000;73(876):1252–9.

[26] Kodama K, Higashiyama M, Yokouchi H, et al. Natural history of pure ground-glass opacity after long-term follow-up of more than 2 years. Ann Thorac Surg 2002;73(2):386–92.

[27] Kakinuma R, Ohmatsu H, Kaneko M, et al. Progression of focal pure ground-glass opacity detected by low-dose helical computed tomography screening for lung cancer. J Comput Assist Tomogr 2004; 28(1):17–23.

[28] Kodama K, Higashiyama M, Yokouchi H, et al. Prognostic value of ground-glass opacity found in small lung adenocarcinoma on high-resolution CT scanning. Lung Cancer 2001;33(1):17–25.

[29] Kondo T, Yamada K, Noda K, et al. Radiologic-prognostic correlation in patients with small pulmonary adenocarcinomas. Lung Cancer 2002;36(1): 49–57.

[30] Suzuki K, Asamura H, Kusumoto M, et al. Early peripheral lung cancer: prognostic significance of ground glass opacity on thin-section computed tomographic scan. Ann Thorac Surg 2002;74(5): 1635–9.

[31] Takamochi K, Nagai K, Yoshida J, et al. Pathologic N0 status in pulmonary adenocarcinoma is predictable by combining serum carcinoembryonic antigen level and computed tomographic findings. J Thorac Cardiovasc Surg 2001;122(2):325–30.

[32] Ohde Y, Nagai K, Yoshida J, et al. The proportion of consolidation to ground-glass opacity on high resolution CT is a good predictor for distinguishing the population of non-invasive peripheral adenocarcinoma. Lung Cancer 2003;42(3):303–10.

[33] Higashiyama M, Kodama K, Yokouchi H, et al. A novel test of the surgical margin in patients with lung cancer undergoing limited surgery: lavage cytologic technique. J Thorac Cardiovasc Surg 2000; 120(2):412–3.

[34] Yamato Y, Tsuchida M, Watanabe T, et al. Early results of a prospective study of limited resection for bronchioloalveolar adenocarcinoma of the lung. Ann Thorac Surg 2001;71(3):971–4.

[35] Watanabe S, Watanabe T, Arai K, et al. Results of wedge resection for focal bronchioloalveolar carcinoma showing pure ground-glass attenuation on computed tomography. Ann Thorac Surg 2002; 73(4):1071–5.

[36] Yamada S, Kohno T. Video-assisted thoracic surgery for pure ground-glass opacities 2 cm or less in diameter. Ann Thorac Surg 2004;77(6):1911–5.

[37] Libby DM, Smith JP, Altorki NK, et al. Managing the small pulmonary nodule discovered by CT. Chest 2004;125(4):1522–9.

ELSEVIER
SAUNDERS

Thorac Surg Clin 17 (2007) 203–215

THORACIC
SURGERY
CLINICS

Open Lobectomy for Patients with Stage I Non–Small Cell Lung Cancer

Shawn S. Groth, MD*, Michael A. Maddaus, MD

*Department of Surgery, University of Minnesota Medical School, MMC 207,
420 Delaware Street SE, Minneapolis, MN 55455, USA*

As the number one overall cause of cancer-related death, lung cancer, whose most common type is non–small cell lung cancer (NSCLC), is a leading public health concern in the United States. Of the estimated 174,470 people in the United States who were diagnosed with lung cancer in 2006 [1], about 18% (31,400 people) had stage I disease [2]. The average 5-year survival rate for stage I NSCLC patients exceeds 65% with appropriate therapy [3–5]. The 5-year survival rate is 0%, however, for untreated patients (median survival, 17 months) [6]. It is paramount that patients with stage I NSCLC undergo proper treatment to maximize their chance of survival. Because stage I tumors are contained within a foci of lung parenchyma, achieving local tumor control by completely resecting the neoplasm is the foundation of treatment [7]. In the 1950s, open lobectomy emerged as the standard of care for treating patients with early stage NSCLC. Since then, despite decades of debate regarding the optimal mode of therapy, lobectomy with mediastinal lymphadenectomy remains the gold standard for treating patients with clinical stage I NSCLC who have sufficient cardiopulmonary reserve, including older patients.

Historical perspective

The operative management of respiratory infectious and inflammatory processes provided much of the initial experience in pulmonary resection and laid the groundwork for modern

thoracic surgical oncology practices [8,9]. In 1901, the first anatomic lobectomy was performed by Gluck [10] for bronchiectasis. The original technique of open lobectomy was crude. Given uncertainty regarding the appropriate management of the lobar bronchus and pulmonary vessels, the first lobectomies were performed as a two-stage operation. In the first operation, a tourniquet was applied to the lobar bronchus and to the pulmonary vessels to induce necrosis of the lung parenchyma, thereby facilitating subsequent lung removal. In the second operation, the bronchus and the vessels were ligated en masse. With time, surgical techniques improved. In 1912, the first modern dissection lobectomy for lung cancer was performed by Davies [11]. Unfortunately, the patient died of empyema 8 days later, which hindered acceptance of lobectomy as a therapeutic option for lung cancer.

Widespread use of lobectomy was further delayed by the promising results obtained by surgeons with other pulmonary resections. In 1932, Graham and Singer [12] successfully performed a pneumonectomy for lung cancer in a 40-year-old obstetrician. For the next two decades, pneumonectomy became the standard of care for lung cancer patients. Nonetheless, interest in lobectomy to treat early stage lung cancer persisted, and the technique for performing the operation was perfected. Brunn [13] departed from the tradition of performing a two-stage lobectomy and introduced the concept of a one-stage procedure. Applying the principles that had been developed for pneumonectomy, Blades and Kent [14] described the technique of individual ligation of the lobar bronchus and each of the pulmonary vessels. Not until the 1950s, however, when

* Corresponding author.
E-mail address: groth015@umn.edu (S.S. Groth).

Churchill and colleagues [15] demonstrated long-term survival after lobectomy for patients with early stage, peripheral lung cancer was lobectomy widely accepted as the standard of care.

Although some surgeons were investigating the use of pneumonectomy and lobectomy, other surgeons were exploring the use of sublobar resection to treat patients with small, peripheral, early stage NSCLC. In the 1860s, Penn [16] performed the first partial pulmonary resection for cancer. As the surgical techniques and as the understanding of pulmonary anatomy improved, anatomic sublobar resection emerged. In 1939, the first anatomic segmentectomy for a patient with bronchiectasis was described [17]. It soon emerged as a therapeutic option for patients with early stage peripheral lung cancer [18]. In 1973, Jensik and colleagues [19] reported a 56.4% actuarial 5-year survival rate in patients with stage I NSCLC undergoing segmentectomy for curative intent; ever since, controversy has existed regarding whether lobectomy or segmentectomy is the more appropriate operation for treating early stage lung cancer, especially in patients who have small peripheral tumors or who are older.

Selection of patients for open lobectomy

The anatomic location of a stage I tumor may suggest that lobectomy is both technically feasible and oncologically appropriate, yet the patient must also have sufficient cardiopulmonary reserve to undergo the operation with an acceptable risk of perioperative morbidity and mortality. All stage I NSCLC patients who are potential candidates for lobectomy must undergo a comprehensive preoperative assessment of their cardiopulmonary function.

Such assessment should include a thorough preoperative history and physical examination, with specific attention paid to signs and symptoms of cardiopulmonary compromise. Several standardized indices, such as metabolic equivalent tests [20] and the Duke Activity Status Index [21], have been established, but a simple review of systems provides an essential, noninvasive means of assessing a patient's functional capacity and stratifying his or her risk of perioperative morbidity and mortality. For instance, a patient who reports an inability to walk four blocks or to climb two flights of stairs without symptomatic limitation has a significantly increased risk of developing perioperative cardiovascular complications [22]. Ancillary studies are a critical adjunct,

but should not supplant the clinician's general assessment of physiologic fitness.

Given the relatively high incidence of perioperative arrhythmias and concomitant cardiovascular disease, a preoperative electrocardiogram should be obtained for all lobectomy candidates [23]. Depending on the presence and severity of clinical predictors of perioperative cardiovascular complications, such as coronary artery disease, heart failure, arrhythmias, valvular disease, diabetes mellitus, and chronic renal insufficiency, additional noninvasive (myocardial perfusion scans, echocardiograms) or invasive (coronary angiography) studies may be required [20].

In addition to evaluating cardiovascular fitness, a patient's pulmonary fitness should also be assessed. A baseline assessment of arterial gas exchange is important for future comparison and provides prognostic information. Specifically, preoperative hypoxemia, defined as an arterial oxygen saturation of less than 90% at rest, is associated with an increased risk of postoperative complications [24]. Despite being historically quoted as an exclusion criterion for pulmonary resection, hypercapnia, defined as a carbon dioxide partial pressure greater than 45 mm Hg, is not an independent risk factor for perioperative complications; it does, however, indicate a need for further physiologic testing [25].

Pulmonary function tests (PFTs) also provide essential information regarding the ability of a patient to tolerate lobectomy with an acceptable risk of perioperative morbidity and mortality. A postbronchodilator forced expiratory volume in 1 second (FEV_1) of at least 1.5 L is considered a safe lower limit for lobectomy candidates; in the absence of interstitial lung disease or excessive dyspnea with exertion, such a volume indicates that further testing is unnecessary [26]. Unfortunately, the literature that stratified perioperative risk was based on absolute values (rather than a normalized percentage) of FEV_1, making it difficult unconditionally to apply a lower limit value of 1.5 L to female patients, older patients, and patients of smaller stature, all of whom may tolerate lobectomy even if their baseline FEV_1 is less than 1.5 L [25]. In patients with either radiographic evidence of, or a known history of, interstitial lung disease or in those who have undue dyspnea on exertion, the diffusion capacity of the lung for carbon monoxide (D_{LCO}) should be assessed, even if the FEV_1 is at least 1.5 L. In patients who have an FEV_1 less than 1.5 L, an FEV_1 less than 80% of the predicted value, or a D_{LCO} less than 80% of the predicted value, the percent predicted postoperative FEV_1 and D_{LCO} should be determined [25]. Patients with a percent predicted postoperative FEV_1 or a percent predicted postoperative D_{LCO} less than 40% are at an increased risk for perioperative complications and require formal cardiopulmonary exercise testing to determine their maximal oxygen consumption (VO_2 max) [25]. Although the threshold has been debated, a VO_2 max of 15 mL/kg/min or greater is indicative of sufficient cardiopulmonary reserve. A VO_2 max less than 15 mL/kg/min is associated with an increased risk of perioperative complications. The care of such patients should be discussed at a multidisciplinary conference and may be limited to nonoperative tumor management [26].

Poor cardiopulmonary function may preclude a patient from undergoing lobectomy, yet age alone should not. Lung cancer primarily affects people over 50, a significant number of whom are over 70 [1]. As the longevity of the general population increases, an increasing number of patients over 70 have lung cancer. The age-adjusted incident rates for patients over 65 increased by over 50% from 1975 (about 250 per 100,000 person-years) to 2003 (about 350 per 100,000 person-years) [2]. An estimated 1 in 16 men and 1 in 24 women age 70 and older developed lung cancer in 2006 [1]. Many older patients, undeservedly so, are denied the choice of a potentially curative operation. According to a study conducted at the Dartmouth Hitchcock Medical Center, only 6% of patients 80 and older with early stage NSCLC underwent surgical resection at that institution [27]. Associated comorbidities may have precluded some older patients from undergoing resection, and others may have refused intervention; nonetheless, a significant proportion were likely denied an operation, because of the erroneous assumption that older patients' postoperative life expectancy is too short or that their quality of life would be impaired. On the contrary, the life expectancy of a 70 year old is 14.7 years, and of an 80 year old, 8.8 years [28]. Furthermore, a 75-year-old individual will likely spend about 60% of the rest of his or her life living independently [29]. The mean survival time of older patients who do not undergo surgical resection is 6 to 12 months [30], as compared with a median survival time of 54 months after resection for stage I NSCLC [31]. A significant number of person-years are lost if physiologically fit older patients are denied an operation. Because the physiologic age and the chronologic age of a patient are often

not synchronous, the appropriateness of surgery must be assessed on an individual basis.

Studies comparing open lobectomy with sublobar resection

Nonrandomized retrospective cohort studies

Because stage I tumors are confined within a foci of lung parenchyma, the goal of a pulmonary resection for stage I NSCLC is to obtain local control of the neoplasm, thereby preventing future tumor dissemination and optimizing the patient's chance for long-term survival. Patients with untreated stage I NSCLC, albeit an early stage neoplasm, have a 5-year survival rate of less than 5% [32,33] (median survival, 12 months [34]). If untreated, even seemingly insignificant stage I tumors that are less than 15 mm have a 90% mortality rate [35]. Radiation and chemotherapy, alone or in combination, offer little additional benefit. Several observational studies have demonstrated a significant survival advantage in NSCLC patients who undergo complete surgical resection, however, whether lobectomy for patients with adequate cardiopulmonary function or a lesser resection for patients with multiple comorbidities and insufficient cardiopulmonary reserve (Table 1) [7,36,37]. The choice of operation, however, is crucial.

Sublobar resection, either wedge resection or anatomic segmentectomy, has been used increasingly as an alternative treatment for patients with stage I NSCLC who lack sufficient pulmonary reserve to tolerate an anatomic lobectomy [38–44]. Several retrospective cohort studies have compared the operative mortality rate, the local recurrence rate, and the 5-year survival rate of sublobar resection with open lobectomy patients (Table 2). Those studies demonstrated higher local recurrence rates after sublobar resection (7.2%–33.9%) than open lobectomy (1.1%–13.3%) [40–44]. Two studies, although noting a trend in favor of lower local recurrence rates after lobectomy, did not demonstrate a statistically significant difference between the two groups, possibly because of a lack of statistical power [42,43]. In assessing the results of those studies, the differences in local recurrence rates are especially noteworthy because the group that underwent sublobar resection (versus standard open lobectomy) tended to have smaller tumors [44]. It is known that local recurrence rates are directly related to the size of the tumor [45]. If lobectomy

Table 1
5-year survival rates following complete surgical resection of stage I non–small cell lung cancer

Author and reference	Study period	Stage[a]	Number of patients	5-year survival
Mountian [7]	1975–1988	pT1N0M0	511	67
		pT2N0M0	549	57
Inoue et al [36]	1980–1993	pT1N0M0	480	80
		pT2N0M0	271	65
Jassem et al [37]	1991–1995	pT1NI0M0	51	66
		pT2N0M0	220	53

Abbreviation: p, pathologic stage.
[a] Stage by TNM classification [7].

and sublobar resection offered equivalent results as some investigators contend, one would have anticipated lower local recurrence rates after sublobar resection on the basis of smaller tumors in that cohort. On the contrary, higher recurrence rates were noted after sublobar resection.

In addition to lower local recurrence rates, those studies suggested a survival advantage after open lobectomy. More favorable cancer-free survival rates, likely the result of differences in local recurrence rates, were achieved after lobectomy (92%) as compared with segmentectomy (75%) or wedge resection (42%) [43]. Some investigators contend that cancer-free survival often does not correlate with overall survival. As a whole, however, the aforementioned series also demonstrated better overall survival rates after open lobectomy (versus sublobar resection).

A few investigators have failed to show a difference in survival rates between the two operations. Their results, however, should be interpreted with reservation. Hoffmann and Ransdell's [38] series demonstrated a 5-year survival rate of 25% after open lobectomy, a rate that was not significantly different from the 5-year survival rate after wedge resection. The patients in their series were treated in the 1960s and 1970s, however, before many of the current advances in perioperative patient care and in critical care, as evidenced by their 5.4% operative mortality rate for patients undergoing lobectomy. Another two studies [39,41] showed no significant difference in the survival rate for patients undergoing lobectomy versus sublobar resection, yet about 25% of patients in each group analyzed in Errett's and coworkers [39] series were not staged. It is conceivable that a significant proportion of patients in either the lobectomy or the sublobar resection cohort may have had more advanced disease than was perceived, which would lead to biased results. Furthermore, the series by Errett

and coworkers [39] and by Pastorino and coworkers [41] do not provide information on the number of lymph nodes that were removed. Because the number of lymph nodes sampled during resection of node-negative NSCLC has important implications for survival [46], insufficient lymph node dissections may have led to lower than expected survival rates in their patients who underwent lobectomy.

Except for three studies just discussed [38,39,41], the remainder of the aforementioned series demonstrated that relatively physiologically fit patients who underwent lobectomy had a more favorable 5-year survival rate (49%–77%), as compared with patients with poor cardiopulmonary reserve who underwent sublobar resection (33%–69%) [39–44]. Patients who underwent sublobar resection tended to be older and tended to have more comorbidities, so these results were likely confounded by differences in the general health of the patients and by differences in tumor size. Simply on the basis of their general state of health, it is not surprising that patients with poor cardiopulmonary reserve who underwent a sublobar resection had a worse 5-year survival rate than physiologically fit patients who underwent a lobectomy [47]. Indeed, in patients who underwent sublobar resection, non–cancer-related deaths were more likely [42].

The aforementioned studies demonstrated that relatively physiologically fit patients who underwent open lobectomy for stage I NSCLC had better local recurrence rates, better cancer-free survival rates, and better overall 5-year survival rates, as compared with patients with poor cardiopulmonary reserve who underwent sublobar resection. Because of the significant differences between the two cohorts, however, the results are difficult to interpret and are not generalizable. This group of studies failed to answer satisfactorily the question of whether or

Table 2
Sublobar resection in stage I non-small cell lung cancer patients without adequate cardiopulmonary reserve versus open lobectomy

Author and reference	Study period	Stage[a]	Sublobar resection										Open lobectomy			
			Wedge resection			Segmentectomy			Aggregate				Number of patients	% Local recurrence	% 5-year survival	% Operative mortality
			Number of patients	% Local recurrence	% 5-year survival	Number of patients	% Local recurrence	% 5-year survival	Number of patients	% Local recurrence	% 5-year survival	% Operative mortality				
Hoffmann and Ransdell [38]	1965–1977	Stage I	33	NR	26[f]							0	112	NR	25[f]	5.4
Erreett et al [39]	1965–1982	Stage I	100	NR	69[c,f]	13	NR	NR				3[f]	97	NR	75[e,f]	2.1[f]
Martini et al [40]	1973–1983	pStage I	49	NR	NR				62	33.9	59	0	511	1.1	77[b]	2.3
Pastorino et al [41]	1971–1988	Stage I							61	8.2	55[f]	0	411	5	49[f]	3
Landreneau et al [42]	1989–1994	pStage Ia	42[c]	24[f]	58							0[f]	117	9[f]	70	3[f]
			60[d]	16[f]	65											
Miller et al [43]	1980–1999	Stage I (T <1 cm)	13	30.8	27	12	8.3[f]	57[f]	25	28[f]	33	4	71	13.3[f]	71[f]	4
El-Sherif et al [44]	1990–2003	Stage I	122	NR	NR	85	NR	NR	207	7.2	40	1.4[f]	577	4.2	54	2.6[f]

Abbreviations: NR, not reported; p, pathologic stage.

[a] Stage by TNM Classification [7].

[b] Survival rate as an aggregate of survival for lobectomy, bilobectomy, and pneumonectomy.

[c] Open wedge resection.

[d] Video-assisted thoracoscopic wedge resection.

[e] 6-Year survival rate.

[f] Results not statistically significant ($P > .05$) versus same outcome in other group.

not sublobar resection and open lobectomy offer equivalent outcomes in patients with sufficient physiologic reserve to tolerate a lobectomy.

Consequently, based on the results of Jensik's and coworkers report [19], several investigators explored the use of anatomic segmentectomy as a possible equivalent alternative to open lobectomy in patients with stage I NSCLC with sufficient cardiopulmonary fitness to tolerate lobectomy (Table 3). Except for the series by Read and colleagues [48], these retrospective cohort studies showed a trend toward lower local recurrence rates after open lobectomy (1.3%–4.9%) than after segmentectomy (2.2%–22.7%) [4,5,45], although the results were not uniformly statistically significant [4,5]. It is likely that the higher recurrence rates after open lobectomy in the series by Read and colleagues [48] are caused by the nonrandomized nature of their study design and by their routine use of lobectomy before the establishment of modern staging techniques [7]. It is conceivable that a number of patients in their series who underwent a lobectomy for purported stage I disease were understaged. The lack of significant differences in local recurrence rates in the studies by Kodama and colleagues [4] and by Koike and colleagues [5] may be caused by small sample sizes or by the difference in tumor sizes: the group that underwent anatomic segmentectomy tended to have smaller tumors, which inherently have lower recurrence rates; a statistically significant difference in local recurrence rates may have been detected if both cohorts had been more closely matched in terms of tumor size.

Except for the series by Warren and Faber [45], the remainder of the studies listed in Table 3 demonstrated no significant differences between the 5-year survival rate after lobectomy (74%–90.1%) versus segmentectomy (84%–93%) [4,5,48]. Because the choice of operation was left to the discretion of the surgeon, it is possible that the lack of a statistically significant difference was caused by selection bias. Indeed, the cohort of patients who were chosen to undergo segmentectomy had statistically significantly smaller tumors than those who underwent lobectomy [4,5,45]. In addition to its correlation with local recurrence rates, it has been well-documented that tumor size has important implications for the survival rate of patients with NSCLC [7,49]. Even among patients with T1 disease, smaller tumors portend a better prognosis [45]. Consequently, the survival rate after sublobar resection may not accurately reflect the results that would be obtained if tumor size in

each group was equivalent. Furthermore, given the concern that segmentectomy patients may require closer postoperative observation, surgeons may have devoted more time to their care and long-term surveillance, leading to additional bias.

Because of the high likelihood of bias and confounding, the aforementioned comparative studies lack sufficient validity to establish whether open lobectomy or segmentectomy offers lower local recurrence rates and higher survival rates in stage I NSCLC patients who have sufficient cardiopulmonary reserve.

Randomized controlled trial

The best available evidence regarding the optimal technique for resecting stage I NSCLC was published by the Lung Cancer Study Group [3]. In that prospective, multi-institutional, randomized clinical trial, patients with stage I NSCLC were deemed eligible for inclusion if they had sufficient cardiopulmonary function to tolerate lobectomy. At the time of thoracotomy, enrolled patients were confirmed to have peripheral, pathologic stage T1N0M0 NSCLC. They were subsequently randomized to undergo either open lobectomy or sublobar resection (wedge resection or anatomic segmentectomy). Between February 1982 and November 1988, 276 patients were randomized. Of those, 247 (125 who underwent lobectomy and 122 who underwent sublobar resection) were eligible for analysis [3]. This clinical trial dispelled the theoretical advantages of sublobar resection and provided evidence supporting its theoretical disadvantages, thereby establishing open lobectomy as the standard of care.

One supposed theoretical advantage of sublobar resection was a reduction in perioperative morbidity and mortality. Except for six patients (5%) in the trial's lobectomy group who required mechanical ventilation for more than 24 hours postoperatively, however, perioperative morbidity and mortality did not significantly differ between the two groups [3].

Another supposed theoretical advantage of sublobar resection is preservation of pulmonary function. To provide objective evidence to explore this hypothesis, the trial investigators examined postoperative PFT results. Of the 60% of patients who completed PFTs at 6 months, those in the sublobar resection (versus lobectomy) group had significantly greater preservation of FEV_1, forced vital capacity, maximum midexpiratory flow rate, and maximum voluntary ventilation. At 12 to 18

Table 3
Sublobar resection in stage I non–small cell lung cancer patients with adequate cardiopulmonary reserve versus open lobectomy

Author and reference	Study period	Stage[a]	Sublobar resection										Open lobectomy			
			Wedge resection			Segmentectomy			Aggregate								
			Number of patients	% Local recurrence	% 5-year survival	Number of patients	% Local recurrence	% 5-year survival	Number of patients	% Local recurrence	% 5-year survival	% Operative mortality	Number of patients	% Local recurrence	% 5-year survival	% Operative mortality
Read et al [48]	1966–1988	Stage Ia				107	4.4	~84[c]				3.5	131	11.5	~74[c]	2.3
Warren and Faber [45]	1980–1988	pStage I				66	22.7	~43[b]				1.5	103	4.9	~67[b]	1.9
Kodoma et al [4]	1985–1996	pStage Ia				46	2.2[c]	93[c]				0	77	1.3[c]	88[c]	0
Koike et al [5]	1992–2000	Stage Ia	14	NR	NR	60	NR	NR	74	2.7[c]	89.1[c]	0	159	1.3[c]	90.1[c]	0

Abbreviations: NR, not reported; p, pathologic stage.

[a] Stage by TNM Classification [7].

[b] Results not statistically significant for tumors <3 cm.

[c] Results not statistically significant versus same outcome in other group (*P* >.05).

months, however, based on the PFT results of 66% of the trial participants, these differences decreased, except for FEV_1. This information is not available for all of the study participants, which diminishes the statistical validity of the results. Nonetheless, these results suggest that, contrary to previous conjecture, there is no significant difference between lobectomy and sublobar resection in terms of long-term preservation of pulmonary function [3].

One supposed theoretical disadvantage of sublobar resection is the potential for higher local recurrence rates. Indeed, the trial found a threefold increase in local recurrence rates after wedge resection and a 2.4-fold increase in local recurrence rates after segmentectomy (versus lobectomy). Of note, tumor size, even if less than 1 cm, did not affect local recurrence rates; the association between sublobar resection and higher local recurrence rates persisted [3]. Because it is known that the cause of death in NSCLC patients is frequently not related to malignancy [47], cancer recurrence is the salient indicator of treatment failure [50]. Although other investigators who conducted nonrandomized studies have argued that segmentectomy is an appropriate operation for patients with stage I tumors less than 10 or 20 mm [51–53], the higher level of evidence of the Lung Cancer Study Group trial demonstrating lower recurrence rates after lobectomy (versus sublobar resection) established open lobectomy as the more efficacious operation.

The reason for higher recurrence rates after sublobar resection is a matter of conjecture. One possible explanation is the inadequate clearance of intralobar lymphatics with a lesser resection. Given the potential for nonsequential lymph node metastasis in NSCLC [54] and for direct metastasis to the mediastinal lymph nodes [55], failure adequately to clear the tumor from the intralobar lymphatics may result in higher recurrence rates. Another potential cause for higher local recurrence rates is synchronous lung cancer, which has an overall incidence rate of 0.4% to 16% in NSCLC patients [56,57]. One study of lobectomy specimens reported a 6.3% incidence of synchronous cancer that had evaded detection by preoperative chest radiograph [58]. Furthermore, bronchioloalveolar carcinoma is often associated with occult high-grade atypical hyperplasia, which cannot be detected before pathologic examination of the surgical specimen and which progresses to invasive carcinoma [59]. Because the Lung Cancer

Study Group used chest radiographs to stage participants, a significant number of occult synchronous tumors or foci of microscopic high-grade atypical hyperplasia may have evaded removal during sublobar resection, thereby allowing these additional lesions to progress to clinically apparent recurrent disease.

Another supposed theoretical disadvantage of sublobar resection was the possibility of lower long-term survival rates. Indeed, by a one-sided statistical analysis, trial patients undergoing sublobar resection had a 30% increase in their overall mortality rate and a 50% increase in their cancer death rate [3]. Surprisingly, stage I NSCLC patients who undergo open lobectomy do not achieve 100% cancer-free survival. Possible explanations include their increased risk of developing metachronous tumors (as compared with the general population) [60–62], to the higher local recurrence rates and worsening survival rates with increasing tumor size (even among T1 stage tumors) [43,53,63–66], to differences in tumor biology [67,68], or to understaging because of undetected micrometastasis [51,69] or satellite metastasis [58].

The results of the aforementioned randomized trial must be interpreted with caution. Because of constraints in accrual time and in subsequent follow-up time, the authors justified the use of a one-sided significance level of 0.10 to maximize the power to detect a potential benefit of lobectomy. Establishing the significance level at 0.10 (rather than the traditional, arbitrary level of 0.05) increased the probability of type I error (ie, the false-positive conclusion that there is a difference in outcome between lobectomy and sublobar resection when there is no difference). The authors were concerned that the trial results could be detrimental to the care of future stage I NSCLC patients unless the potential for type II error (ie, the false-negative conclusion that there is not a difference in outcome between lobectomy and sublobar resection when there is a difference) was reduced [3]. Despite these limitations, this is the most rigorously designed trial addressing the question of whether lobectomy or sublobar resection is the most appropriate operation for patients with stage I NSCLC. Until future prospective randomized clinical trials provide evidence to the contrary, an open lobectomy should be considered the standard of care for treating stage I NSCLC in patients who have sufficient physiologic reserve to tolerate the operation.

Results of open lobectomy in older patients

Open lobectomy should also be considered the standard of care for treating older patients (≥70) with stage I NSCLC who have sufficient cardiopulmonary reserve. In carefully selected older patients, perioperative mortality rates of 0% to 3% can be achieved [54,70–75]. Series with higher mortality rates should be interpreted with caution. Several studies reporting high (14%–19%) mortality rates were published before the institution of modern advances in perioperative patient care and the associated decrease in perioperative mortality rates [76,77]. Furthermore, many studies describing the outcomes of older patients after pulmonary resection included patients with stage I to III disease. Because advanced (versus early) stage is associated with worse survival rates, the overall survival rates of older patients in these studies were likely diluted by the intrinsic lower survival rates in patients with stage III NSCLC. Furthermore, in part because patients with more advanced disease were included in these studies, as many as 10% to 50% of patients in these series underwent pneumonectomy, which inherently has a higher mortality rate in all age groups, as compared with lobectomy and lesser resection [78,79].

The rate of perioperative complications in older patients after any pulmonary resection is 13% to 65% [31,54,71–75,77,80–83]. The few studies that delineated complication rates by resection type reported morbidity rates of 21% to 44% after lobectomy [31,80,84]. Not surprisingly, older patients have a higher tendency to develop cardiopulmonary complications than do their younger counterparts. Of note, multivariate analyses in most studies demonstrated that age is not independently associated with perioperative morbidity and mortality [70,80,85,86]. Appropriate patient selection, however, is essential, as exemplified in a recent study by Matsuoka and colleagues [74]: 40 octogenarians with stage I to III disease had a mortality rate of 0% and a complication rate of 20% after resection. Their results are consistent with published mortality [3,5,44] and complication [87] rates in recent series of predominantly younger patients. Open lobectomy can be performed with acceptable morbidity and mortality rates in older patients.

Older patients who undergo lobectomy have a distinct survival advantage [30]. As compared with those who receive palliative therapy (median survival, less than 8 months [77]), appropriately selected older patients with stage I NSCLC have a 5-year survival rate of 45% to 79% [31,54,71–74,81,82,84,86,88], which is comparable with the 5-year survival rate in recent series involving predominantly younger patients [3,5,44]. The Surveillance Epidemiology and End Results (SEER) Program database was used in a recent study to explore survival trends in older patients following pulmonary resection [89]. In a post hoc analysis, investigators reported that the survival advantage of lobectomy (versus sublobar resection) was lost in patients older than 71 [89]. The overall study results incorporated the outcomes of patients with stage II disease, who inherently have a worse prognosis than those with stage I NSCLC. The survival advantage after lobectomy may have persisted through all age groups, if only stage I patients had been included. In addition, because older patients tend to undergo fewer diagnostic procedures than their younger counterparts, a significant number of patients in the SEER database may be understaged. Furthermore, the investigators provided no information regarding associated comorbidities (which is a limitation of the SEER database) or on the number of mediastinal lymph nodes that were assessed; both factors have a significant impact on survival rates [46,47,90–92]. Their analysis should be interpreted cautiously.

Finally, older patients with stage I NSCLC can undergo open lobectomy without compromising their quality of life. Some clinicians may contend that older patients are likely to spend their last years in an assisted living environment and that an operation hastens their loss of independent living. On the contrary, in a study of octogenarians who underwent pulmonary resection for NSCLC, more than 94% did not require convalescence at a transitional care unit and were discharged directly to their homes [82]. Other clinicians may argue that lobectomy is detrimental to an older patient's long-term postoperative pulmonary function and quality of life. Sullivan and colleagues [93] provided evidence to the contrary, demonstrating no significant difference in postoperative PFTs or subjective quality of life (as determined using Karnofsky scores) between older (≥70) and younger patients 1 year following lobectomy. Both younger and older patients were able to live and to function postoperatively at the same capacity that they had enjoyed before undergoing lobectomy [93].

Mediastinal lymphadenectomy: a critical adjunct to open lobectomy

Complete mediastinal lymph node dissection is an important adjunct to open lobectomy. Assessment of the mediastinal lymph nodes is an essential component of accurate tumor staging, which enables clinicians to offer NSCLC patients the most appropriate therapy. The method by which mediastinal lymph nodes are assessed is crucial. Because patients who undergo mediastinal lymphadenectomy have better survival rates [90] than those who undergo lymph node sampling [91], complete mediastinal lymph node dissection should not be supplanted by less thorough techniques. Importantly, patient survival after resection for NSCLC is directly associated with the number of lymph nodes removed [46,91,92]. Although the optimal number has yet to be determined, an analysis of the SEER database by Ludwig and colleagues [46] indicated that 11 to 16 lymph nodes should be removed. Differences in survival rates in patients who underwent lobectomy in the aforementioned cohort studies may be caused, in part, by whether or not the mediastinal lymph nodes were assessed (either by lymph node sampling or by formal lymphadenectomy) and by how many lymph nodes were removed. Many of the surgeons likely removed an insufficient number of lymph nodes.

A recent national patient care survey by the American College of Surgeons provides evidence in favor of this conjecture. Investigators noted that mediastinal lymph nodes were assessed in only 46.6% of nearly 11,700 patients with NSCLC who underwent pulmonary resection [94]. Indeed, much improvement is needed in the care of patients with NSCLC.

Finally, despite concerns to the contrary, complete mediastinal lymphadenectomy adds little morbidity [90,91,95], makes no difference in postoperative length of stay [95], and adds only 15 minutes to the operative time [95]. The role of mediastinal lymphadenectomy in stage I NSCLC is more thoroughly reviewed elsewhere in this issue.

Summary

Until additional multi-institutional, randomized, controlled trials provide evidence to the contrary, open lobectomy with mediastinal lymphadenectomy should be considered the gold standard for treating patients with stage I NSCLC with sufficient cardiopulmonary reserve, including older patients. It is the operation with which alternative pulmonary resections, including video-assisted thoracoscopic lobectomy and sublobar resection, should be compared. In treating stage I NSCLC patients, sublobar resection should be reserved for patients with inadequate physiologic reserve to tolerate lobectomy and for those enrolled in clinical trials.

Acknowledgments

The authors are indebted to Mary E. Knatterud, PhD, for her invaluable assistance in the preparation of this manuscript.

References

[1] Jemal A, Siegel R, Ward E, et al. Cancer statistics, 2006. CA Cancer J Clin 2006;56(2):106–30.
[2] Surveillance, Epidemiology, and End Results (SEER) Program. Available at: http://www.seer.cancer.gov/. SEER*Stat Database: Incidence–SEER 17 Regs Public-Use, Nov 2005 Sub (1973-2003 varying), National Cancer Institute, DCCPS, Surveillance Research Program, Cancer Statistics Branch, released April 2006.
[3] Ginsberg RJ, Rubinstein LV. Randomized trial of lobectomy versus limited resection for T1 N0 non-small cell lung cancer. Lung Cancer Study Group. Ann Thorac Surg 1995;60(3):615–22; [discussion: 613–22].
[4] Kodama K, Doi O, Higashiyama M, et al. Intentional limited resection for selected patients with T1 N0 M0 non-small-cell lung cancer: a single-institution study. J Thorac Cardiovasc Surg 1997;114(3): 347–53.
[5] Koike T, Yamato Y, Yoshiya K, et al. Intentional limited pulmonary resection for peripheral T1 N0 M0 small-sized lung cancer. J Thorac Cardiovasc Surg 2003;125(4):924–8.
[6] Vrdoljak E, Mise K, Sapunar D, et al. Survival analysis of untreated patients with non-small-cell lung cancer. Chest 1994;106(6):1797–800.
[7] Mountain CF. Revisions in the International System for Staging Lung Cancer. Chest 1997;111(6):1710–7.
[8] Lowson D. A case of pneumonectomy. Br Med J 1893;1:1152–4.
[9] MacEwen W. The Cavendish lecture on some points in the surgery of the lung. Br Med J 1906;2:1–7.
[10] Gluck T. Die entwickelung de lungenchirurgie. Verhandlungen des Kongresses Fur Innere Medizin 1901;19:478–92.
[11] Davies HM. Recent advances in the surgery of the lung and pleura. Br J Surg 1913;1:228–58.

[12] Graham EA, Singer JJ. Successful removal of the entire lung for carcinoma of the bronchus. JAMA 1933;101(18):1371–4.

[13] Brunn H. Surgical principles underlying one stage lobectomy. Arch Surg 1929;18(1):490–515.

[14] Blades B, Kent EM. Individual ligation techniques for lower lobe lobectomy. J Thorac Surg 1940; 10(1):84–101.

[15] Churchill ED, Sweet RH, Sutter L, et al. The surgical management of carcinoma of the lung: a study of cases treated at the Massachusetts General Hospital from 1930–1950. Surgery 1950;20:349–65.

[16] Penn J. Chirgurie des poumons. Discussion Ranc Chir Proc Verh Paris 1895;9:72.

[17] Churchill ED, Belsey R. Segmental pneumonectomy in bronchiectasis the lingula segment of the left upper lobe. Ann Surg 1939;109(2):481–99.

[18] Hewlett TH, Gomez AC, Aronstam EM, et al. Bronchiolar carcinoma of the lung: review of 39 patients. J Thorac Cardiovasc Surg 1964;48:614–24.

[19] Jensik RJ, Faber LP, Milloy FJ, et al. Segmental resection for lung cancer: a fifteen-year experience. J Thorac Cardiovasc Surg 1973;66(4): 563–72.

[20] Eagle KA, Berger PB, Calkins H, et al. ACC/AHA guideline update for perioperative cardiovascular evaluation for noncardiac surgery: executive summary. A report of the American College of Cardiology/American Heart Association Task Force on Practice Guidelines (Committee to Update the 1996 Guidelines on Perioperative Cardiovascular Evaluation for Noncardiac Surgery). Circulation 2002;105(10):1257–67.

[21] Hlatky MA, Boineau RE, Higginbotham MB, et al. A brief self-administered questionnaire to determine functional capacity (the Duke Activity Status Index). Am J Cardiol 1989;64(10):651–4.

[22] Reilly DF, McNeely MJ, Doerner D, et al. Self-reported exercise tolerance and the risk of serious perioperative complications. Arch Intern Med 1999; 159(18):2185–92.

[23] Conti VR, Ware DL. Cardiac arrhythmias in cardiothoracic surgery. Chest Surg Clin N Am 2002;12(2): 439–60.

[24] Ninan M, Sommers KE, Landreneau RJ, et al. Standardized exercise oximetry predicts postpneumonectomy outcome. Ann Thorac Surg 1997;64(2):328–32; [discussion: 323–332].

[25] Beckles MA, Spiro SG, Colice GL, et al. The physiologic evaluation of patients with lung cancer being considered for resectional surgery. Chest 2003;123(1 Suppl):105S–14S.

[26] British Thoracic Society; Society of Cardiothoracic Surgeons of Great Britain and Ireland Working Party. BTS guidelines: guidelines on the selection of patients with lung cancer for surgery. Thorax 2001;56(2):89–108.

[27] Nugent WC, Edney MT, Hammerness PG, et al. Non-small cell lung cancer at the extremes of age: impact on diagnosis and treatment. Ann Thorac Surg 1997;63(1):193–7.

[28] US National Center for Health Statistics, Vital Statistics of the United States, annual. National Vital Statistics Report. vol 53.

[29] Katz S, Branch LG, Branson MH, et al. Active life expectancy. N Engl J Med 1983;309(20):1218–24.

[30] Harviel JD, McNamara JJ, Straehley CJ. Surgical treatment of lung cancer in patients over the age of 70 years. J Thorac Cardiovasc Surg 1978;75(6): 802–5.

[31] Brock MV, Kim MP, Hooker CM, et al. Pulmonary resection in octogenarians with stage I nonsmall cell lung cancer: a 22-year experience. Ann Thorac Surg 2004;77(1):271–7.

[32] Salomaa ER, Liippo K, Taylor P, et al. Prognosis of patients with lung cancer found in a single chest radiograph screening. Chest 1998;114(6):1514–8.

[33] Flehinger BJ, Kimmel M, Melamed MR. The effect of surgical treatment on survival from early lung cancer: implications for screening. Chest 1992; 101(4):1013–8.

[34] Jazieh AR, Kyasa MJ, Sethuraman G, et al. Disparities in surgical resection of early-stage non-small cell lung cancer. J Thorac Cardiovasc Surg 2002;123(6): 1173–6.

[35] Henschke CI, Wisnivesky JP, Yankelevitz DF, et al. Small stage I cancers of the lung: genuineness and curability. Lung Cancer 2003;39(3):327–30.

[36] Inoue K, Sato M, Fujimura S, et al. Prognostic assessment of 1310 patients with non-small-cell lung cancer who underwent complete resection from 1980 to 1993. J Thorac Cardiovasc Surg 1998; 116(3):407–11.

[37] Jassem J, Skokowski J, Dziadziuszko R, et al. Results of surgical treatment of non-small cell lung cancer: validation of the new postoperative pathologic TNM classification. J Thorac Cardiovasc Surg 2000;119(6):1141–6.

[38] Hoffmann TH, Ransdell HT. Comparison of lobectomy and wedge resection for carcinoma of the lung. J Thorac Cardiovasc Surg 1980;79(2):211–7.

[39] Errett LE, Wilson J, Chiu RC, et al. Wedge resection as an alternative procedure for peripheral bronchogenic carcinoma in poor-risk patients. J Thorac Cardiovasc Surg 1985;90(5):656–61.

[40] Martini N, Bains MS, Burt ME, et al. Incidence of local recurrence and second primary tumors in resected stage I lung cancer. J Thorac Cardiovasc Surg 1995;109(1):120–9.

[41] Pastorino U, Valente M, Bedini V, et al. Limited resection for stage I lung cancer. Eur J Surg Oncol 1991;17(1):42–6.

[42] Landreneau RJ, Sugarbaker DJ, Mack MJ, et al. Wedge resection versus lobectomy for stage I (T1 N0 M0) non-small-cell lung cancer. J Thorac Cardiovasc Surg 1997;113(4):691–8; [discussion: 698–700].

[43] Miller DL, Rowland CM, Deschamps C, et al. Surgical treatment of non-small cell lung cancer 1 cm or

less in diameter. Ann Thorac Surg 2002;73(5): 1545–50; [discussion: 1541–50].

[44] El-Sherif A, Gooding WE, Santos R, et al. Outcomes of sublobar resection versus lobectomy for stage I non-small cell lung cancer: a 13-year analysis. Ann Thorac Surg 2006;82(2):408–15; [discussion: 406–15].

[45] Warren WH, Faber LP. Segmentectomy versus lobectomy in patients with stage I pulmonary carcinoma: five-year survival and patterns of intrathoracic recurrence. J Thorac Cardiovasc Surg 1994; 107(4):1087–93; [discussion: 1084–93].

[46] Ludwig MS, Goodman M, Miller DL, et al. Postoperative survival and the number of lymph nodes sampled during resection of node-negative non-small cell lung cancer. Chest 2005;128(3):1545–50.

[47] Battafarano RJ, Piccirillo JF, Meyers BF, et al. Impact of comorbidity on survival after surgical resection in patients with stage I non-small cell lung cancer. J Thorac Cardiovasc Surg 2002;123(2): 280–7.

[48] Read RC, Yoder G, Schaeffer RC. Survival after conservative resection for T1 N0 M0 non-small cell lung cancer. Ann Thorac Surg 1990;49(3):391–8; [discussion: 399–400].

[49] Lopez-Encuentra A, Duque-Medina JL, Rami-Porta R, et al. Staging in lung cancer: is 3 cm a prognostic threshold in pathologic stage I non-small cell lung cancer? A multicenter study of 1,020 patients. Chest 2002;121(5):1515–20.

[50] Thomas P, Rubinstein L. Cancer recurrence after resection: T1 N0 non-small cell lung cancer. Lung Cancer Study Group. Ann Thorac Surg 1990;49(2): 242–6; [discussion: 246–7].

[51] Ohta Y, Oda M, Wu J, et al. Can tumor size be a guide for limited surgical intervention in patients with peripheral non-small cell lung cancer? Assessment from the point of view of nodal micrometastasis. J Thorac Cardiovasc Surg 2001;122(5): 900–6.

[52] Okada M, Yoshikawa K, Hatta T, et al. Is segmentectomy with lymph node assessment an alternative to lobectomy for non-small cell lung cancer of 2 cm or smaller? Ann Thorac Surg 2001;71(3):956–60; [discussion: 961].

[53] Okada M, Nishio W, Sakamoto T, et al. Effect of tumor size on prognosis in patients with non-small cell lung cancer: the role of segmentectomy as a type of lesser resection. J Thorac Cardiovasc Surg 2005; 129(1):87–93.

[54] Ishida T, Yokoyama H, Kaneko S, et al. Long-term results of operation for non-small cell lung cancer in the elderly. Ann Thorac Surg 1990;50(6):919–22.

[55] Riquet M, Hidden G, Debesse B. Direct lymphatic drainage of lung segments to the mediastinal nodes: an anatomic study on 260 adults. J Thorac Cardiovasc Surg 1989;97(4):623–32.

[56] Ferguson MK. Synchronous primary lung cancers. Chest 1993;103(4 Suppl):398S–400S.

[57] McElvaney G, Miller RR, Muller NL, et al. Multicentricity of adenocarcinoma of the lung. Chest 1989;95(1):151–4.

[58] Saito Y, Sato M, Sagawa M, et al. Multicentricity in resected occult bronchogenic squamous cell carcinoma. Ann Thorac Surg 1994;57(5):1200–5.

[59] Koga T, Hashimoto S, Sugio K, et al. Lung adenocarcinoma with bronchioloalveolar carcinoma component is frequently associated with foci of high-grade atypical adenomatous hyperplasia. Am J Clin Pathol 2002;117(3):464–70.

[60] Thomas PA Jr, Rubinstein L. Malignant disease appearing late after operation for T1 N0 non-small-cell lung cancer. The Lung Cancer Study Group. J Thorac Cardiovasc Surg 1993;106(6): 1053–8.

[61] Rice D, Kim HW, Sabichi A, et al. The risk of second primary tumors after resection of stage I non-small cell lung cancer. Ann Thorac Surg 2003; 76(4):1001–7; [discussion: 1007–8].

[62] Pasini F, Verlato G, Durante E, et al. Persistent excess mortality from lung cancer in patients with stage I non-small-cell lung cancer, disease-free after 5 years. Br J Cancer 2003;88(11):1666–8.

[63] Jackman RJ, Good CA, Clagett OT, et al. Survival rates in peripheral bronchogenic carcinomas up to four centimeters in diameter presenting as solitary pulmonary nodules. J Thorac Cardiovasc Surg 1969;57(1):1–8.

[64] Wisnivesky JP, Yankelevitz D, Henschke CI. The effect of tumor size on curability of stage I non-small cell lung cancers. Chest 2004;126(3):761–5.

[65] Ramacciato G, Paolini A, Volpino P, et al. Modality of failure following resection of stage I and stage II non-small cell lung cancer. Int Surg 1995;80(2): 156–61.

[66] Thomas P, Doddoli C, Thirion X, et al. Stage I non-small cell lung cancer: a pragmatic approach to prognosis after complete resection. Ann Thorac Surg 2002;73(4):1065–70.

[67] Pechet TT, Carr SR, Collins JE, et al. Arterial invasion predicts early mortality in stage I non-small cell lung cancer. Ann Thorac Surg 2004;78(5):1748–53.

[68] Kondo D, Yamada K, Kitayama Y, et al. Peripheral lung adenocarcinomas: 10 mm or less in diameter. Ann Thorac Surg 2003;76(2):350–5.

[69] D'Cunha J, Herndon JE II, Herzan DL, et al. Poor correspondence between clinical and pathologic staging in stage 1 non-small cell lung cancer: results from CALGB 9761, a prospective trial. Lung Cancer 2005;48(2):241–6.

[70] Pagni S, McKelvey A, Riordan C, et al. Pulmonary resection for malignancy in the elderly: is age still a risk factor? Eur J Cardiothorac Surg 1998;14(1): 40–4; [discussion: 44–5].

[71] Bernet F, Brodbeck R, Guenin MO, et al. Age does not influence early and late tumor-related outcome for bronchogenic carcinoma. Ann Thorac Surg 2000;69(3):913–8.

[72] Port JL, Kent M, Korst RJ, et al. Surgical resection for lung cancer in the octogenarian. Chest 2004;126(3):733–8.

[73] Aoki T, Tsuchida M, Watanabe T, et al. Surgical strategy for clinical stage I non-small cell lung cancer in octogenarians. Eur J Cardiothorac Surg 2003;23(4):446–50.

[74] Matsuoka H, Okada M, Sakamoto T, et al. Complications and outcomes after pulmonary resection for cancer in patients 80 to 89 years of age. Eur J Cardiothorac Surg 2005;28(3):380–3.

[75] Ciriaco P, Zannini P, Carretta A, et al. Surgical treatment of non-small cell lung cancer in patients 70 years of age or older. Int Surg 1998;83(1):4–7.

[76] Weiss W. Operative mortality and five year survival rates in patients with bronchogenic carcinoma. Am J Surg 1974;128(6):799–804.

[77] Kirsh MM, Rotman H, Bove E, et al. Major pulmonary resection for bronchogenic carcinoma in the elderly. Ann Thorac Surg 1976;22(4):369–73.

[78] Thomas P, Sielezneff I, Ragni J, et al. Is lung cancer resection justified in patients aged over 70 years? Eur J Cardiothorac Surg 1993;7(5):246–50; [discussion: 241–50].

[79] Naunheim KS, Kesler KA, D'Orazio SA, et al. Lung cancer surgery in the octogenarian. Eur J Cardiothorac Surg 1994;8(9):453–6.

[80] Sioris T, Salo J, Perhoniemi V, et al. Surgery for lung cancer in the elderly. Scand Cardiovasc J 1999;33(4):222–7.

[81] Shirakusa T, Tsutsui M, Iriki N, et al. Results of resection for bronchogenic carcinoma in patients over the age of 80. Thorax 1989;44(3):189–91.

[82] Pagni S, Federico JA, Ponn RB. Pulmonary resection for lung cancer in octogenarians. Ann Thorac Surg 1997;63(3):785–9.

[83] Osaki T, Shirakusa T, Kodate M, et al. Surgical treatment of lung cancer in the octogenarian. Ann Thorac Surg 1994;57(1):188–92; [discussion: 183–92].

[84] Massard G, Moog R, Wihlm JM, et al. Bronchogenic cancer in the elderly: operative risk and long-term prognosis. Thorac Cardiovasc Surg 1996;44(1):40–5.

[85] Morandi U, Stefani A, Golinelli M, et al. Results of surgical resection in patients over the age of 70 years with non small-cell lung cancer. Eur J Cardiothorac Surg 1997;11(3):432–9.

[86] Sherman S, Guidot CE. The feasibility of thoracotomy for lung cancer in the elderly. JAMA 1987;258(7):927–30.

[87] Deslauriers J, Ginsberg RJ, Piantadosi S, et al. Prospective assessment of 30-day operative morbidity for surgical resections in lung cancer. Chest 1994;106(6 Suppl):329S–30S.

[88] Yamamoto K, Padilla Alarcon J, Calvo Medina V, et al. Surgical results of stage I non-small cell lung cancer: comparison between elderly and younger patients. Eur J Cardiothorac Surg 2003;23(1):21–5.

[89] Mery CM, Pappas AN, Bueno R, et al. Similar long-term survival of elderly patients with non-small cell lung cancer treated with lobectomy or wedge resection within the surveillance, epidemiology, and end results database. Chest 2005;128(1):237–45.

[90] Doddoli C, Aragon A, Barlesi F, et al. Does the extent of lymph node dissection influence outcome in patients with stage I non-small-cell lung cancer? Eur J Cardiothorac Surg 2005;27(4):680–5.

[91] Lardinois D, Suter H, Hakki H, et al. Morbidity, survival, and site of recurrence after mediastinal lymph-node dissection versus systematic sampling after complete resection for non-small cell lung cancer. Ann Thorac Surg 2005;80(1):268–74; [discussion: 265–74].

[92] Gajra A, Newman N, Gamble GP, et al. Effect of number of lymph nodes sampled on outcome in patients with stage I non-small-cell lung cancer. J Clin Oncol 2003;21(6):1029–34.

[93] Sullivan V, Tran T, Holmstrom A, et al. Advanced age does not exclude lobectomy for non-small cell lung carcinoma. Chest 2005;128(4):2671–6.

[94] Little AG, Rusch VW, Bonner JA, et al. Patterns of surgical care of lung cancer patients. Ann Thorac Surg 2005;80(6):2051–6; [discussion: 2056].

[95] Allen MS, Darling GE, Pechet TT, et al. Morbidity and mortality of major pulmonary resections in patients with early-stage lung cancer: initial results of the randomized, prospective ACOSOG Z0030 trial. Ann Thorac Surg 2006;81(3):1013–9; [discussion: 1019–20].

ELSEVIER
SAUNDERS

Thorac Surg Clin 17 (2007) 217–221

THORACIC
SURGERY
CLINICS

Role of Lymphadenectomy in the Treatment of Clinical Stage I Non–Small Cell Lung Cancer

Tiziano De Giacomo, MD[a], Federico Venuta, MD[a],
Erino Angelo Rendina, MD[b],*

[a]University of Rome "La Sapienza," Division of Thoracic Surgery, Policlinico Umberto I,
Dipartimento Paride Stefanini, Via le del Policlinico 155, 00161 Rome, Italy
[b]University of Rome "La Sapienza," Division of Thoracic Surgery, Ospedale Sant'Andrea,
Via di Grottarossa 1035, 00189 Rome, Italy

Although surgical resection is considered the gold standard for stage I non–small cell lung cancer (NSCLC), long-term results are unsatisfying because as many as 30% of patients develop local or distant recurrence after complete resection. Possible explanations are the presence of distant micrometastasis at the time of resection or the technique of the bronchopulmonary and mediastinal lymph node dissection (MLND) during the operation.

The ideal extent of MLND during lung cancer surgery has long been controversial among thoracic surgeons and gold standards have not yet been established. In stages I to IIIa NSCLC the options range from simple inspection and palpation of the mediastinum, to systemic sampling, to selective or radical MLND. Also, it still remains unclear whether lobectomy with node sampling is therapeutically equivalent to lobectomy with radical systematic node dissection in small peripheral NSCLC.

The arguments in favor of lymphadenectomy are the improvement of the accuracy of lung cancer staging, the improvement of the indications for subsequent adjuvant therapy, the decrease of locoregional recurrence, and ultimately the improvement of survival. Against MLND plays the unclear advantage in long-term survival, the increase in operative time, blood loss, and postoperative complications.

Extent of lymph node dissection

The first issue to be addressed is the absence of a standardized surgical method for lymph node sampling or dissection, and this point hampers the analysis of the international literature on the argument. Gaer and Goldstraw [1] compared the intraoperative inspection and palpation of resected lymph nodes with the definitive histologic diagnosis demonstrating the surgeon's inability to determine the lymph node involvement without biopsy. Systematic node sampling should be preferred to random sampling. Systematic sampling consists of multiple level, bronchopulmonary, and mediastinal lymph node biopsies.

The concept of lymphadenectomy is even less well defined and only a few papers in the literature have reported detailed data on the number and site of removed lymph nodes. Only recently [2,3], it has been suggested that the quality of lymphadenectomy should be evaluated on the number and level of nodes harvested, although reported cutoff values vary greatly. The Eastern Cooperative Oncology Group in the ECOG 3590 trial defined lymphadenectomy as the procedure that harvests 10 or more nodes in two or more mediastinal stations [4]. Complete mediastinal lymphadenectomy for tumors on the right side requires removing all lymph tissue from an area bounded caudally by the takeoff of the right upper lobe, superiorly by the innominate artery, anteriorly

* Corresponding author.
  E-mail address: erinoangelo.rendina@uniroma1.it
(E.A. Rendina).

1547-4127/07/$ - see front matter © 2007 Published by Elsevier Inc.
doi:10.1016/j.thorsurg.2007.03.008

by the superior vena cava, and posteriorly by the trachea. For tumors on the left side, complete lymphadenectomy includes all lymphatic tissue from the area beneath the phrenic nerve anteriorly and the vagus nerve posteriorly. Superiorly, all lymph tissue to the top of the aortic arch should be removed using as caudal boundary the left mainstem bronchus. Regardless of the tumor side, complete subcarinal, both mainstem bronchi, inferior pulmonary ligament, posterior pericardium, and lobar and interlobar lymph nodes should be removed. Systematic MLND, as practiced by Japanese surgeons [5], is a much more extensive operation including extensive aortic mobilization and dissection of high mediastinal node on the left side and above the subclavian artery on the right side. This procedure requires longer operative time and it is probably associated with higher morbidity. Okada and colleagues [6] recently described the concept of selective mediastinal lymphadenectomy for clinicosurgical stage I NSCLC: dissection of the upper mediastinum for upper lobe tumors but not for lower lobe tumors with intact hilar and lower mediastinal nodes; dissection of the lower mediastinum is not routinely required for an upper lobe tumor with negative nodes at the hilum and in the upper mediastinum. Yoshimasu and colleagues [7] recently have supported the concept of regional MLND: if regional mediastinal lymph nodes (Table 1) are not metastatic, dissection of mediastinal nodes can be stopped at this point.

Sentinel lymph node mapping techniques, extensively studied for melanoma and breast cancer, have been applied more recently to most solid tumors. The safety and efficacy of sentinel lymph node mapping has been documented in patients with lung cancer [8–10]. Its application to lung cancer is still controversial but if it were

Table 1
Lymph node levels for regional and standard mediastinal node dissection

Tumor location	Regional node dissection	Standard node dissection
Right upper lobe	2,3,4	1,2,3,4,7
Right lower lobe	3,7,8	1,2,3,4,7,8,9
Left upper lobe	4,5,7	4,5,6,7
Left lower lobe	4,7,8	4,5,6,7,8

Data from Yoshimasu T, Miyoshi S, Oura S, et al. Limited mediastinal lymph node dissection for non small cell lung cancer according to intra-operative histologic examinations. J Thorac Cardiovasc Surg 2005;130: 433–7.

valid, early stage lung cancer would gain the most benefit, because sentinel lymph node biopsy could reduce the need for systemic MLND [11].

Risks of mediastinal lymph node dissection

Potential risks of lymph node dissection include devitalization of bronchial tree with possible bronchial stump dehiscence and fistula, bleeding, chylothorax, laryngeal nerve palsy, impairment of lymphatic back-flow with pulmonary edema, or acute respiratory distress syndrome. Many surgeons, frightened by these risks, have preferred to proceed with lymph node sampling, consisting of random biopsies at the main nodal stations. Other surgeons have adopted the strategy to identify the sentinel node, using radioisotope, to avoid the potential damage caused by mediastinal dissection in early stage lung cancer [8–10].

The myth of increased complications following formal node dissection is swept away by five prospective randomized trials. Izbicki and associates [12,13], based on 182 patients, demonstrated that the complications of patients undergoing radical lymphadenectomy are equal to those of patients subjected to sampling; and so did the large study on 532 patients from Wu and coworkers [14]. The latter reports an overall morbidity of 5% with no intraoperative deaths. In the MLND group, one patient died of pulmonary edema on the seventh postoperative day for a 30-day mortality of 0.31%. The study from Keller and associates [15], a large prospective multicentric nonrandomized trial based on 373 patients, although not intended to evaluate complications, shows that nodal dissection does not entail increased blood losses or mean operative time when compared with sampling. More recently, Lardinois and coworkers [16] confirmed that there was no significant difference in terms of morbidity, duration of drainage, and hospital stay when comparing sampling with dissection. Doddoli and colleagues [17] showed no difference in complications between sampling and dissection except for left laryngeal nerve palsy, more frequent after lymphadenectomy. Finally, the large multi-institutional study from the American College of Surgeons (ACOSOG Z0030) based on a group of a 1111 patients clearly demonstrates that there is no difference in the incidence of complications; although the operation was prolonged by a median of 15 minutes, no difference in length of hospitalization was observed (Table 2) [18].

Table 2
Mediastinal lymph node dissection does not entail increased complications

Four prospective randomized trials		
Izbicki et al [13]	182 patients	No difference in mortality, complications, chest tube, hospital stay
Wu et al [14]		
Lardinois et al [16]	532 patients	
ACOSOG Z0030 [18]	100 patients	
	1111 patients	
One prospective nonrandomized trial		
Keller et al [15]	373 patients	Equal blood losses and operative time

Impact on staging

Accurate pathologic staging remains a basic recommendation for management of NSCLC, because staging allows one to estimate prognosis and hence to define the most adequate treatment strategy. The hypothesis that a complete lymph node dissection is superior to node sampling for adequate determination of N stage has been validated by different studies. Gajra and colleagues [2] reviewed 442 patients with stage I disease, classified into quartiles according to the number of nodes harvested: less than four, four to six, seven to nine, and more than nine. Corresponding 5-year disease-free survival rates were 47.3%, 72.8%, 76.4%, and 79.1%, respectively. Furthermore, 5-year survival was 61.9% when no station was explored, and 87.6% for four or more stations, confirming that the more nodes resected the more likely is the reality of stage I.

Izbicki and coworkers [13] found that in the sampling group only 4 (17.4%) of 23 patients with N2 disease had more than one level involved, whereas mediastinal dissection results in the detection of multiple N2 disease in 12 (57.2%) of 21 patients. This difference is statistically significant and results in a shorter disease-free and overall survival (Table 3).

In a work from Keller and associates [15] among 222 patients with N2 disease, multiple levels of N2 were documented in 12% of the patients who had sampling and in 30% of patients who underwent dissection ($P = .001$). These two studies demonstrate that MLND identifies significantly more levels of N2 disease, which is an important contribution to the accuracy of staging and is of prognostic significance. The study from Lardinois and coworkers [16], a prospective randomized trial on 100 patients with a very long follow-up, indicates that the disease-free interval in stage I patients is significantly longer

after lymph node dissection than after sampling. Also, in patients with a negative mediastinum, the rate of local recurrence is significantly higher after sampling than after mediastinal dissection. More interesting data have been reported by Wu and colleagues [14] in a randomized trial including 532 patients and comparing sampling with node dissection. As expected, dissection staged more patients with N2 disease (sampling, 42% stage I and 28% stage IIIa; dissection, 24% stage I and 48% stage IIIa). More recently, Massard and coworkers [19] published a multicentric cross-sectional study on 208 patients with operable NSCLC. Before lung resection mediastinum was explored and lymph node sampling was performed; subsequently, the usual lymph node dissection was accomplished. Node sampling adequately identified 31 (52%) out of 60 N2 patients and multilevel N2 was discovered at sampling in 10 (40%) out 25 patients.

Impact on survival

Although there are an increasing number of studies suggesting that lymph node dissection

Table 3
Mediastinal lymph node dissection improves staging and local control

Izbicki et al [13]	182 patients	$P < .001$
Multiple N2 disease revealed by SS	17.4%	
Multiple N2 disease revealed by MLND	57.2%	
Keller et al [15]	373 patients	$P = .001$
Multiple N2 disease revealed by SS	12%	
Multiple N2 disease revealed by MLND	30%	

Abbreviations: MLND, mediastinal lymph node dissection; SS, systematic sampling.

Table 4
Mediastinal lymph node dissection improves survival

Keller et al [15]	
Median survival SS	29.2 mo
Median survival MLND	57.7 mo
Wu et al [14]	
Median survival SS	34 mo
Median survival MLND	59 mo

Abbreviations: MLND, mediastinal lymph node dissection; SS, systematic sampling.

improves survival, this issue is not yet completely clarified, especially for early stage lung cancer. Two important large prospective studies with a long follow-up and one meta-analysis of systematic lymph node dissection demonstrate that dissection has a significant survival advantage over sampling. The study from Keller and associates [15] shows that median survival was 29.2 months for patients who had undergone sampling and 57.5 months for those who had dissection. The survival advantage was limited, however, to patients with right lung tumors (24.5 versus 66.4 months; $P < .001$). The large prospective randomized study from Wu and associates [14] demonstrates a median survival of 34 months in the sampling group and 59 months in the dissection group. When the patients are divided by stage, the authors noted that there is a statistically significant difference in stage I (57.49% versus 82.16% 5-year survival); only marginal difference in stage II (34.05% versus 50.42% 5-year survival); and a statistically significant difference in stage IIIA (6.18% versus 26.98%). In a recent meta-analysis, the same group analyzed four trials for a total of 997 patients; they found that there is a significant improvement in 5-year survival and that the overall odds ratio for death is decreased by 0.33 for mediastinal dissection versus sampling in resectable NSCLC (Table 4) [20].

On the contrary, Sugi and associates [21] conducted a randomized prospective trial comparing sampling with systematic mediastinal node dissection in 115 patients with clinical T1N0 tumors that were less than 2 cm in diameter. Mediastinal lymph node involvement was found in 13% of each study group, and no difference in recurrence patterns or survival was found.

Summary

It has been proved with acceptable certainty that MLND does not increase complications in lung cancer surgery and improves the accuracy of staging. This applies to lung cancer at all resectable stages. As far as survival is concerned, statistically significant differences have been suggested by some authors and are more evident for early stages. Stage I NSCLC, a local disease, may profit from lymph node dissection, a procedure that can effectively control local tumor, reduce local recurrence, and improve long-term survival.

References

[1] Gaer JAR, Goldstraw P. Intraoperative assessment of nodal staging at thoracotomy for carcinoma of the bronchus. Eur J Cardiothorac Surg 1990;4: 207–10.

[2] Gajra A, Newman N, Gamble P, et al. Effects of number of lymph nodes sampled on outcome in patients with stage I non small cell lung cancer. J Clin Oncol 2003;21:1029–33.

[3] Wu IC, Lin CFJ, Hsu WH, et al. Long-term results of pathological stage I non small cell lung cancer: validation of using the number of totally removed lymphnodes as a staging control. Eur J Cardiothorac Surg 2003;24:994–1001.

[4] Keller SM, Adak S, Wagner H, et alThe Eastern Cooperative Oncology Group. Mediastinal lymphadenectomy in non small cell lung cancer: effectiveness in patients with or without nodal micrometastases—results of a preliminary study. Eur J Cardiothorac Surg 2002;21:520–6.

[5] Oda M, Watanabe Y, Shimizu J, et al. Extent of mediastinal node metastasis in clinical stage I non small cell lung cancer: the role of systematic nodal dissection. Lung Cancer 1998;22:23–30.

[6] Okada M, Sakamoto T, Yuki T, et al. Selective mediastinal lymphadenectomy for clinico-surgical stage I non small cell lung cancer. Ann Thorac Surg 2006;81:1028–33.

[7] Yoshimasu T, Miyoshi S, Oura S, et al. Limited mediastinal lymph node dissection for non small cell lung cancer according to intra-operative histologic examinations. J Thorac Cardiovasc Surg 2005;130: 433–7.

[8] Nomori H, Watanabe K, Ohtsuka T, et al. In vivo identification of sentinel lymph nodes for clinical stage I non small cell lung cancer for abbreviation of mediastinal lymph node dissection. Lung Cancer 2004;46:49–55.

[9] Melfi FM, Chella A, Menconi GF, et al. Intraoperative radioguided sentinel lymph node biopsy in non small cell lung cancer. Eur J Cardiothorac Surg 2003;23:214–20.

[10] Lyptay MJ, Masters GA, Winchester DJ, et al. Intraoperative radioisotope sentinel lymph node mapping in non small cell lung cancer. Ann Thorac Surg 2000;70:384–9.

[11] Sugi K, Kaneda Y, Sudoh M, et al. Effect of radioisotope sentinel node mapping in patients with

cT1N0M0 lung cancer. J Thorac Cardiovasc Surg 2003;126:568–73.

[12] Izbicki JR, Thetter O, Habekost M, et al. Radical systematic lymphadenectomy in non small cell lung cancer. Br J Surg 1994;81:229–35.

[13] Izbicki JR, Passlick B, Karg O, et al. Impact of radical systematic mediastinal lymphadenectomy on tumor staging in lung cancer. Ann Thorac Surg 1995; 59(1):209–14.

[14] Wu Y, Huang Z, Wang S, et al. A randomized trial of systemic nodal dissection in resectable non small cell lung cancer. Lung Cancer 2002;36:1–6.

[15] Keller SM, Adak S, Wagner H, et al. Mediastinal lymph node dissection improves survival in patients with stages II and IIIa non small cell lung cancer. Ann Thorac Surg 2000;70:358–66.

[16] Lardinois D, Suter H, Hakki H, et al. Morbidity survival and site of recurrence after mediastinal lymph node dissection versus systematic sampling after complete resection for non small cell lung cancer. Ann Thorac Surg 2005;27:680–5.

[17] Doddoli C, Aragon A, Barlesi F, et al. Does the extent of lymph node dissection influence outcome in patients with stage I non small cell lung cancer? Eur J Cardiothorac Surg 2005;27:680–5.

[18] Allen MS, Darling GE, Pechet TT, et al. Morbidity and mortality of major pulmonary resections in patients with early stage lung cancer: initial results of the randomized, prospective ACOSOG Z0030 trial. Ann Thorac Surg 2006;81:1013–9.

[19] Massard G, Ducrocq X, Kochtkova EA, et al. Sampling or node dissection for intraoperative staging of lung cancer: a multicentric cross-sectional study. Eur J Cardiothorac Surg 2006;30:164–7.

[20] Yang H, Wu Y, Chen G. A meta-analysis of systematic lymph node dissection in NSCLC. [ASCO Annual Meeting Proceedings]. J Clin Oncol 2004;22: 7190.

[21] Sugi K, Nawata K, Fujita N, et al. Systematic lymph node dissection for clinically diagnosed peripheral non small cell lung cancer less than 2 cm in diameter. World J Surg 1998;22:290–5.

THORACIC
SURGERY
CLINICS

ELSEVIER
SAUNDERS

Thorac Surg Clin 17 (2007) 223–231

Video-Assisted Thoracoscopic Surgery Lobectomy for Stage I Lung Cancer

Ali Mahtabifard, MD, Daniel T. DeArmond, MD,
Clark B. Fuller, MD, Robert J. McKenna, Jr, MD*

*Section of Thoracic Surgery, Department of Cardiothoracic Surgery, Cedars-Sinai Medical Center,
8635 West Third Street, Suite 975W, Los Angeles, CA 90048, USA*

Video-assisted thoracoscopic surgery (VATS) is an appealing alternative to thoracotomy for lobectomy in patients who have stage I lung cancer. The success of laparoscopy in the 1980s and improved endoscopic video systems and endoscopic staplers led thoracic surgeons to apply this technology to the chest cavity. Since the first VATS lobectomy (VL) with anatomic hilar dissection performed in 1992, investigators from around the world have published small series that report the safety and advantages of this approach. This article reviews the current literature of VATS lobectomy for stage I lung cancer.

The worldwide experience with VATS lobectomy for early-stage lung cancer is sufficiently large to compare this procedure with open thoracotomy. VL can be performed safely and provides several benefits. Postoperative pain following VL is significantly less, and patients return to full activity sooner. In addition, some studies document better preservation of pulmonary function. These attributes of VL allow recruitment of older patients and patients with multiple comorbidities that would otherwise have made them unsuitable for conventional open thoracotomy. As such, the momentum to perform minimally invasive pulmonary resections is growing in the field of general thoracic surgery.

Definition of video-assisted thoracoscopic surgery lobectomy

The exact definition of a VATS lobectomy is controversial. The controversies center around rib spreading, instrumentation, and anatomic dissection. Most surgeons agree that a VL should be performed through an incision less than 10 cm long and that the ribs should not be spread. The soft tissue can be held open by a Wietlander retractor so that suctioning in the chest does not expand the lung. Visualization of the chest cavity and the hilum is on the monitor and not through the incision. Some surgeons use standard open instruments, whereas others use disposable, minimally invasive instruments; however, this should not be part of the definition. An absolute is that a VL should be a standard anatomic dissection. Although simultaneous ligation of the hilar structures has been reported [1], it is to be discouraged.

Indications and contraindications

Almost all patients who have stage I non-small cell lung cancer are candidates for VATS lobectomy. In 2005, 94% of 239 lobectomies we performed were by way of VATS. The work-up includes a physiologic evaluation to ensure that there are no medical contraindications, such as poor pulmonary function or severe cardiac disease. We do not obtain cardiac stress testing routinely unless the EKG is abnormal or there is a history of cardiac disease. Pulmonary function tests should predict that the postoperative forced expiratory volume in 1 second (FEV_1) will be at

* Corresponding author.
  E-mail address: mckennar@cshs.org
(R.J. McKenna).

1547-4127/07/$ - see front matter © 2007 Elsevier Inc. All rights reserved.
doi:10.1016/j.thorsurg.2007.03.019

thoracic.theclinics.com

least 40% of predicted. If the pulmonary function test is borderline, the patient may need a quantitative pulmonary perfusion test to determine if the area to be resected has minimal function, so that it can be resected.

Patients also are evaluated to rule out metastatic disease. Specific tests are ordered based upon the patient's symptoms. For example, a brain MRI is ordered only if the patient has headaches or neurologic symptoms. Positron emission tomographic (PET) scans are used to look for nodal or distant metastasis. Mediastinoscopy is performed unless the tumor is clinical stage IA by preoperative PET and CT scans.

Almost all lobectomies for stage I disease can be done with VATS. Box 1 lists the indications and relative contraindications for VATS lobectomy. Except for the inability to tolerate single-lung ventilation, most limitations are due to anatomic considerations. A tumor larger than 6 cm cannot be removed through a VATS incision. Many thoracic surgeons do not feel that they can safely dissect abnormal lymph nodes from pulmonary vessels. Tumors that invade the chest wall or mediastinum require a thoracotomy, but they are not stage I and are not included in this article. We have performed 10 sleeve lobectomies and two bronchoplasties by VATS, so centrally located tumors do not necessarily require a thoracotomy.

Operative technique

Anesthesia and positioning

VATS lobectomy is not an easy operation, and it requires an absolute understanding of thoracic anatomy and mastery of advanced thoracoscopic skills. Single-lung ventilation with a double-lumen endotracheal tube is used almost always.

Box 1. Indications and relative contraindications for video-assisted thoracoscopic surgery lobectomy

Indications
Stage IA and IB cancer
Tumors less than 6 cm

Relative contraindications
Intolerance of single lung ventilation
Tumor size >6 cm
Significant hilar lymphadenopathy
Chest wall or mediastinal involvement

Although some anesthesiologists use CPAP or intermittent ventilation of the lung being operated on, this rarely should be necessary. Intraoperative hypoxia, even in patients with severe emphysema ($FEV_1 < 30\%$), usually is due to poor placement of the double-lumen endotracheal tube and can be corrected by simple adjustment of the tube using bronchoscopy. While under single-lung general anesthesia, the patient is placed in full lateral decubitus position, as for a posterolateral thoracotomy, with a slight posterior tilt. Care is taken to flex the patient fully to prevent the hip from obstructing the movement of the thoracoscope and to maximize the intercostal space opening. The surgeon stands on the anterior side of the patient, and the assistant stands posteriorly. For preemptive analgesia, local anesthetic (0.5% bupivicane with epinephrine) is injected into the intercostal space of the incision, as well as one space above and a few spaces below. Care is taken to infiltrate the inferior border of the ribs without injecting into the intravascular space. This can be done under direct visualization after the thoracoscope is inserted. The goal is to "raise a wheal" just superficial to the endothoracic fascia. This provides an effective intercostal nerve block that can reduce postoperative pain.

Incisions

A 2-cm incision is made in the sixth intercostal space in the midclavicular line and carried into the chest. A finger is inserted through this incision to confirm the lack of adhesions. Next, a 5-mm incision is made in the eighth intercostal space in the midaxillary line, and the chest is entered. Entry into the chest should be angled superiorly and travel over the top of the bottom rib to reduce irritation of the intercostal nerve. The 5-mm port and 5-mm, 30° thoracoscope are placed through this second incision. By placing this incision low in the chest, the best panoramic view of the thoracic cavity is achieved. In addition, the 30° lens allows much greater flexibility for the surgeon to see around structures of the hilum. All other incisions are made directly in the middle of the intercostal space (Fig. 1).

A ring forceps through the midclavicular incision pushes the lung posteriorly to expose the superior pulmonary vein. The 4- to 6-cm utility incision is made directly up from the superior pulmonary vein (generally the fourth intercostal space) for upper lobectomies or one intercostal space lower for middle or lower lobectomies. This

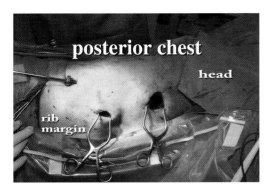

Fig. 1. Patient positioning and location of incisions.

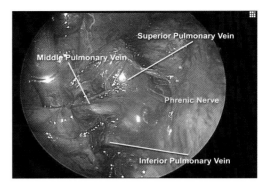

Fig. 2. Pulmonary veins. After incising the pleura over the right hilum, the individual pulmonary veins are clearly identified. Note the location of the phrenic nerve.

incision extends anteriorly from the latissimus muscle. Ribs are not spread, but a Weitlander retractor may be used to hold the soft tissues of the chest wall open for easier passage of instruments and to prevent the lung from expanding when intrathoracic suctioning causes negative pressure in the chest. The hilar structures are easily accessible for dissection through this incision. Often, a 1-cm incision is made in the auscultatory triangle to facilitate dissection and provide further control of the operation, especially when teaching.

Conduct of the operation

With gentle manipulation, all aspects of the lung, and, therefore, all lesions, can be palpated directly through the utility incision. Trocars are not used except for the camera. The entire operation is performed with conventional long instruments that are available in any operating room and are familiar to the thoracic surgeon. If present, adhesions are taken down with the long electrocautery, and the entire lung is mobilized fully. Next, dissection of the hilar structures is begun with visualization on the monitor. The clarity and magnification that are afforded by modern-day optics provide a comprehensive view of the hilar structures. We previously reported the technical details of how to perform the various lobectomies and direct the reader to the appropriate reference [2]. Suffice it to say that the pulmonary vein, artery, and bronchus are individually identified, dissected, isolated, and stapled (Ethicon, Cincinnati, Ohio) (Figs. 2–6). Articulation of the stapler is unnecessary because proper placement of the incisions at the outset provides optimal angles. The incisions that offer the best

angles for stapling various structures are shown in Table 1.

The fissure is then completed and once the lobe is completely disconnected, it is placed in a Lap Sac (Cook Urological, Spencer, Indiana) and brought out through the utility incision. Although the fissure usually is completed after the vessels and the bronchus are transected, one should not hesitate to complete the fissure earlier if this maneuver provides better access to the vessels or the bronchus. A largely fused fissure is not a contraindication to VATS lobectomy, and, in fact, should not alter the conduct of the operation in any way.

A complete mediastinal lymph node dissection is then done thoracoscopically, which was outlined in earlier publications [2,3]. The chest is irrigated, and the bronchial stump is checked for an air leak. Two 28F chest tubes are placed, and

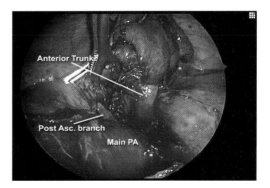

Fig. 3. VATS right upper lobectomy. After opening the fissure and dissection of the right pulmonary artery, the branches of the right pulmonary artery (PA) are individually identified and stapled. Asc, ascending.

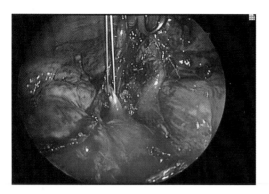

Fig. 4. VATS right upper lobectomy. The posterior ascending branch of the right PA is encircled with a tie and then stapled.

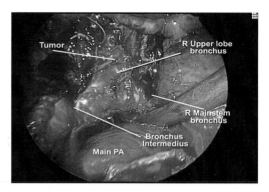

Fig. 6. VATS right upper lobectomy. The right mainstem bronchus, right upper lobe (RUL) bronchus, and bronchus intermedius are clearly identified. The RUL bronchus can now be divided with a tissue stapler.

the incisions are closed. A segmentectomy can be performed for T1 tumors in patients who cannot tolerate a lobectomy.

Results of video-assisted thoracoscopic surgery lobectomy

Since February 1992, we have performed more than 1500 VATS lobectomies. In 2005, we reported our results for the first 1100 in the largest series to date of VATS lobectomies [4], and those results are discussed here. This series included 595 (54.1%) women and 505 men (45.9%), with a mean age of 71.2 years (range, 16–94 years); 160 patients were at least 80 years of age.

The resections performed are seen in Table 2. The pathologic diagnoses for the 1100 resections include primary lung cancer (1015 patients), benign diseases (53 patients; Table 3), metastatic

disease (27 patients), and lymphoma (5 patients, including two cases of mucosa associated lymphoid tissue). Table 4 shows the pathologic diagnoses for the patients with tumors. The preoperative and postoperative staging for the 1015 cases of primary lung cancer are seen in Table 5. Cases were staged as IIIB and IV postoperatively if there were satellite lesions (T4 tumors) or if a metastasis was found in another lobe (M1).

Hospital course

The mean length of stay (LOS) was 4.78 days, and the median LOS was 3 days. On the first postoperative day, 32 (2.9%) patients were discharged; an additional 194 (17.6%) patients were discharged on the second postoperative day

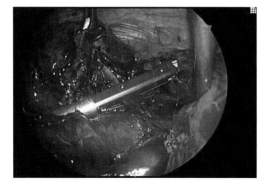

Fig. 5. VATS right upper lobectomy. The vascular stapler is brought through the posterior incision, and the anterior trunk of the right PA is stapled.

Table 1
Recommended incisions for stapler placement

Incision	Structure stapled
Posterior incision	Superior pulmonary vein
	Upper lobe anterior trunk
	Middle lobe artery and vein
	Left upper lobe bronchus
Utility incision	Minor fissure
	Right upper lobe bronchus
Midclavicular incision	Inferior pulmonary vein
	Upper lobe anterior trunk
	Major fissure
	Additional left upper lobe arteries
	Lower lobe arteries
	Lower lobe bronchus

Table 2
The variety of anatomic pulmonary resections that were done with video-assisted thoracoscopic surgery

Right upper lobectomy	403
Right middle lobectomy	92
Right lower lobectomy	158
Pneumonectomy	14
Segmentectomy	19
Sleeve lobectomy	3
Bilobectomy	18
Bilateral lobectomy	1
Left upper lobectomy	279
Left lower lobectomy	113

(Table 6). As the experience with VATS lobectomies grows in our thoracic surgical unit, the LOS is being reduced even further. In our latest report of fast-tracking patients who have undergone VATS lobectomy, the median LOS is less than 3 days, and 46% of our patients are being discharged by postoperative day 2. We usually do not check postoperative chest radiographs or laboratory tests unless clinically indicated, and most of the chest tubes are removed on postoperative day 1 or 2.

Mortality and morbidity

There were no intraoperative deaths. There were nine (0.8%) postoperative deaths due to the following causes: respiratory failure (3), pulmonary embolus (3), myocardial infarct (2), and venous mesenteric infarct (1).

Table 3
The benign diagnoses for which 53 patients underwent video-assisted thoracoscopic surgery lobectomy

Diagnosis	Number of cases
Granuloma	12
Bronchiectasis	11
Abscess	8
Hamartoma	7
UIP	6
BOOP	2
Fungus ball	2
Paraganglioma	1
PA aneurysm	1
Sclerosing hemangioma	1
Sequestration	1
Amyloid	1

Abbreviations: BOOP, bronchiolitis obliterans; PA, pulmonary artery; UIP, usual interstitial pneumonitis.

Table 4
The pathologic type of tumors resected

Pathology	Number of cases
Adenocarcinoma	641
Squamous cell	135
BAC	52
Carcinoid	51
AD SQ	47
Large cell	43
NSCL	30
Small cell	6
Sarcoma	3
Mucoepidermoid	3

Abbreviations: AD SQ, adenocarcinoma–squamous cell carcinoma; BAC, bronchioalveolar carcinoma; NSCL, unclassified non-small cell cancer.

Nine hundred and thirty-two (84.7%) patients had no complications. The remaining 168 patients had one or more of the complications listed in Table 7. Forty-five patients (4.1%) required a blood transfusion during their postoperative course. Thirteen patients were readmitted to the hospital for the following reasons: wound infection (2), chest pain (2), pneumonia (1), dyspnea (1), empyema (1), fall/neck fracture (1), myocardial infarction (1), and subcutaneous air (4).

Conversion to thoracotomy

In 28 (2.5%) cases, the procedure was converted to a thoracotomy for the following reasons: evaluation of the tumor to determine the optimal resection (7), bleeding (7), excessive adhesions (4), size of the tumor precluding removal through the utility incision (3), sleeve resection (3), chest wall invasion (3), and to repair a bronchus that had been injured during double-lumen endotracheal tube placement (1).

Table 5
The preoperative and postoperative staging of the 1015 patients who underwent video-assisted thoracoscopic surgery anatomic resections for primary lung cancer

Stage	Preoperative	Postoperative
1A	653 (59.4%)	561 (51%)
1B	313 (28.5%)	248 (22.5%)
2A	14 (1.3%)	50 (4.5%)
2B	12 (0.9%)	28 (2.5%)
3A	23 (2.2%)	109 (9.9%)
3B	0	17 (1.5%)
4	0	2 (0.2%)

Table 6
The number of patients who were discharged on postoperative days 1 though 10

POD	Patients (N)	Percent
1	32	2.9%
2	194	17.6%
3	294	26.7%
4	198	18%
5	117	10.6%
6	64	5.8%
7	57	5.2%
8	34	3.1%
9	17	1.5%
10	12	1.1%
>10	71	6.5%

Abbreviation: POD, postoperative day.

Survival

The Kaplan-Meier survival for the patients who underwent VATS anatomic resections for primary lung cancer is shown (see Fig. 1).

Table 7
Complications after video-assisted thoracoscopic surgery anatomic resections

None	932
Air leak	56
AF	32
Serous drainage	14
Readmit	13
Pneumonia	13
SQ	12
MI	10
Empyema	4
BPF	3
Atelectasis	2
UTI	2
GI	2
Splenectomy	1
Pericarditis	1
Stroke	1
ARDS	1
TIA	1

Nine hundred and thirty-two (84.7%) patients experienced no complications. Some patients experienced more than one complication.

Abbreviations: ARDS, acute respiratory distress syndrome; AF, atrial fibrillation; air leak, air leak lasting ≥7 days; BPF, broncho-pleural fistula; GI, gastrointestinal complications {Ogilvie's syndrome, GI bleed}; MI, myocardial infarction; serous drainage, serous drainage requiring chest tube drainage >7 days; SQ, subcutaneous air requiring reinsertion of chest tube or subcutaneous catheters; TIA, transient ischemic attack; UTI, urinary tract infection.

Published data about video-assisted thoracoscopic surgery lobectomy

Published series of VL show that the procedure is being performed around the world [5–14]; however, only an overwhelming minority of lobectomies is being performed by way of VATS (<10% is our best guess). Although there are many reasons for this lack of widespread dissemination, the main factor is probably that most thoracic surgeons are still uncomfortable with this technique. As more residents are trained to perform VL, as the technology improves, and as the overall momentum toward minimally invasive surgery continues, more VLs will be performed; one day it may become the standard of care for the treatment of early-stage lung cancer.

Evidence-based medicine suggests that VL may have advantages over a lobectomy by thoracotomy. Opponents of the procedure believe that a VL is unsafe, an incomplete cancer operation, and offers no advantage over a thoracotomy for lobectomy. Although there is no large randomized, prospective series to compare the two approaches, published data suggest that those concerns are unfounded. In fact, the VATS approach is safe and has advantages. In the largest published experience with VL, we showed that the procedure can be performed safely and with some apparent advantages over a thoracotomy [4].

Bleeding with video-assisted thoracoscopic surgery

One area of concern is the risk for blood loss with a VATS procedure. In a nonrandomized study, Sugiura and colleagues [15] compared 22 patients who underwent a lobectomy by VATS with 22 patients who underwent thoracotomy. There was no significant difference in the average operative time (150 ± 126 minutes versus 300 ± 192 minutes), and the blood loss was significantly less (P = .0089) for the VATS group. In a nonrandomized comparison, Demmy and Curtis [16] also found that VL was associated with significantly decreased blood loss compared with open thoracotomy. Therefore, VL performed by experienced VATS surgeons does not seem to carry an increased risk for bleeding.

Another area of concern is the ability to deal with significant bleeding if it should occur during a VATS procedure. This is a valid concern and a logical issue to address. VL is an advanced video procedure and requires mature thoracoscopic skills. To dissect out pulmonary vessels visualized on the monitor is not a skill that all surgeons possess; however, with good judgment and training, major life-threatening hemorrhage should be infrequent. In an international survey of 1578 VLs, there was only one intraoperative death [17]. This was due to a myocardial infarction, not hemorrhage; therefore, the risk for massive hemorrhage seems to be low. In our series [4], only 7 of 1100 cases were converted to an open procedure to control bleeding, and there were no deaths associated with these episodes. The scrub nurse should keep a sponge stick available so that it can be used to apply pressure if bleeding occurs. Once the bleeding is controlled temporarily, the surgeon decides if definitive control can be achieved with VATS or if a thoracotomy is required. With advanced thoracoscopic skills, most vascular injuries can be controlled by way of VATS, and a conversion usually is not necessary.

Hospitalization after video-assisted thoracoscopic surgery lobectomy

Hospitalization seems to be shortened and improved after a VATS procedure. In Demmy and Curtis's [16] nonrandomized series, patients who underwent VATS had shorter hospitalizations (5.3 ± 3.7 days versus 12.2 ± 11.1 days; $P = .02$), shorter chest tube durations (4.0 ± 2.8 days versus 8.3 ± 8.9 days; $P = .06$), and earlier returns to full preoperative activities (2.2 ± 1.0 months versus 3.6 ± 1.0 months; $P < .01$). Pain 3 weeks later was dramatically better for the group that underwent VATS (none or mild: 63% versus 6%; severe: 6% versus 63%; $P < .01$). They concluded that VL is less painful and may offer faster recovery for the frail or high-risk patient. In 2005, 46% of our patients were discharged by postoperative day 2, and the median LOS in our last 300 VLs is 2.93 days. Under the best circumstances, conventional thoracotomies could not yield such results.

Morbidity and mortality after video-assisted thoracoscopic surgery

An important consideration is the overall morbidity and mortality of VL. In a randomized trial from Germany, there were fewer complications after the VATS approach (14.2% versus 50%) [18]. In a nonrandomized comparison of VATS and thoracotomy for lobectomy, Sugiura and colleagues [15] found no difference in the morbidity and mortality. Our experience has shown a paucity of postoperative complications,

including death, compared with historical complication rates. In our latest review [4], almost 85% of our patients experienced no complications, and the mortality was less than 1%.

Pain after video-assisted thoracoscopic surgery

As many studies have shown, postoperative pain is less after a VATS procedure compared with conventional thoracotomy. In a prospective, randomized trial of VATS versus muscle-sparing thoracotomy for lobectomy, Giudicelli and colleagues [19] demonstrated that the postoperative pain was significantly less in the VATS group. Comparing postoperative acute pain in patients who underwent VATS or thoracotomy, Sugiura and colleagues [15] found many factors that favored the VATS group: duration of epidural catheter (3 ± 2 days versus 7 ± 4 days; $P = .0001$), less postoperative narcotic use ($P = .0439$), and the mean frequency of analgesics (14 ± 5 times versus 18 ± 5 times). Walker [20] reported lower visual pain scale, total dose of narcotics, need for additional narcotics, need for intercostal blocks, and sleep disturbances after VATS than a thoracotomy for lobectomy. In addition, there may be a lower incidence of postthoracotomy pain syndrome after VATS than after a thoracotomy [15]. At our center, we do not use epidural catheters for any VATS lobectomy. Patients take oral pain medications in addition to intravenous analgesics postoperatively. Once the chest tubes are removed, most, if not all, patients are transitioned to oral pain medications and discharged with a prescription for oral pain medication. Most patients are off pain medications completely by their first office visit on postoperative day 7.

Postoperative recovery after video-assisted thoracoscopic surgery

Postoperative pulmonary function also seems to be better after VATS than after a thoracotomy. In a nonrandomized comparison of patients who had a lobectomy by a thoracotomy or VATS, postoperative Pao_2, O_2 saturation, peak flow rates, FEV_1, and forced vital capacity on postoperative days 7 and 14 were better for the patients who had undergone the VATS procedure [21]. Patients who undergo VATS have less impairment of pulmonary function and a better 6-minute walk test than do patients who undergo thoracotomy [22].

The short- and long-term quality of life may be better after minimally invasive surgery. For 22 patients who underwent VL and 22 patients who underwent thoracotomy, the time until return to preoperative activity was 2.5 ± 1.7 months with VATS, which was significantly shorter ($P = .0267$) than the 7.8 ± 8.6 months with thoracotomy [15]. VL is associated with significant decreases in shoulder dysfunction compared with thoracotomy [23,24].

Video-assisted thoracoscopic surgery lobectomy as a cancer operation

Although some thoracic surgeons have expressed concerns about the adequacy of VL as a cancer operation, a proper VL should be—and, in the hands of skilled VATS surgeons is—the same operation with the same nodal sampling or dissection that is performed through a thoracotomy. Because a lobectomy should be the same operation by VATS and by thoracotomy, both approaches should be oncologically comparable.

The best measure of any cancer treatment is survival and that should be the ultimate endpoint. Sugi and colleagues [25] found the 5-year survival was 90% and 85% with VATS and thoracotomy, respectively ($P = .74$). Some surgeons have reported exceptional survival after VATS lobectomy: 94.4% at 4 years [26] and 86% (mean, 18.6 months) [1]. Yim and colleagues [27] reported a trend toward improved disease-free survival with VATS resection and suggested that less suppression of immunosurveillance was important to the survival benefit. Others, including our center, have reported survival rates that are the same as those reported with conventionally treated lung cancer: 72% at 5 years [4,28] and 77.9% at 5 years [9]. It seems that a VATS approach does not compromise the survival for patients who have lung cancer.

Summary

The literature shows that, in the hands of experienced thoracoscopic surgeons, VL is a safe operation that offers patients at least comparable complication and survival rates compared with lobectomy by thoracotomy. VL can be performed safely with proven advantages over conventional thoracotomy for lobectomy: smaller incisions, decreased postoperative pain, decreased LOS, decreased chest tube output and duration, decreased blood loss, better preservation of pulmonary function, and earlier return to normal activities. These results are obtained without

sacrificing the oncologic principles of thoracic surgery, and, in fact, the evidence in the literature is mounting that VATS may offer reduced rates of complications and better survival.

References

[1] Lewis RJ, Caccavale RJ. Video-assisted thoracic surgical non-rib spreading simultaneously stapled lobectomy (VATS(n)SSL). Semin Thorac Cardiovasc Surg 1998;10:332.

[2] McKenna RJ Jr. VATS lobectomy with mediastinal lymph node sampling or dissection. Chest Surg Clin N Am 1995;4:223.

[3] McKenna RJ Jr, Fischel RJ. VATS lobectomy and lymph node dissection or sampling in eighty-year-old patients. Chest 1994;106:1902.

[4] McKenna RJ Jr, Houck W, Fuller CB. Video-assisted thoracic surgery lobectomy: experience with 1100 cases. Ann Thorac Surg 2006;81:421.

[5] Kaseda S, Aoki T, Hangai N. Video-assisted thoracic surgery (VATS) lobectomy: the Japanese experience. Semin Thorac Cardiovasc Surg 1998;10:300.

[6] Leschber G, Holinka G, Linder A. Video-assisted mediastinoscopic lymphadenectomy (VAMLA)—a method for systematic mediastinal lymph node dissection. Eur J Card Thorac Surg 2003;24(2):192–5.

[7] Yim APC, et al. Thoracoscopic major lung resections: an Asian perspective. Sem Thorac Cardiovasc Surg 1998;10:326.

[8] Hermansson U, Konstantinov IE, Aren C. Video-assisted thoracic surgery (VATS) lobectomy: the initial Swedish experience. Semin Thorac Cardiovasc Surg 1998;10:285.

[9] Walker WS, Codispoti M, Soon SY, et al. Long-term outcomes following VATS lobectomy for non-small cell bronchogenic carcinoma. Eur J Cardiothorac Surg 2003;23(3):397–402.

[10] Roviaro G, et al. Video-assisted thoracoscopic surgery (VATS) major pulmonary resections: the Italian experience. Semin Thorac Cardiovasc Surg 1998;10:313.

[11] Solaini L, Prusciano F, Bagioni P, et al. Video-assisted thoracic surgery major pulmonary resections. Present experience. Eur J Cardiothorac Surg 2001; 20(3):437–42.

[12] McKenna RJ Jr, et al. VATS lobectomy: the Los Angeles experience. Semin Thorac Cardiovasc Surg 1998;10:321.

[13] Daniels LJ, Balderson SS, Onaitis MW, et al. Thoracoscopic lobectomy: a safe and effective strategy for patients with stage I lung cancer. Ann Thorac Surg 2002;74(3):860–4.

[14] Watanabe A, Osawa H, Watanabe T, et al. Complications of major lung resections by video-assisted thoracoscopic surgery. Jap J Thorac Surg 2003; 56(11):943–8.

[15] Sugiura H, Morikawa T, Kaji M, et al. Long-term benefits for the quality of life after video-assisted thoracoscopic lobectomy in patients with lung cancer. Surg Laparosc Endosc Percutan Tech 1999; 9(6):403–10.

[16] Demmy TL, Curtis JJ. Minimally invasive lobectomy directed toward frail and high-risk patients: a case-control study. Ann Thorac Surg 1999;68(1): 194–200.

[17] Mackinlay TA. VATS Lobectomy: an international survey. Presented at the IVth International Symposium on Thoracoscopy and Video-Assisted Thoracic Surgery. Sao-Paulo (Brazil), May 1997.

[18] Hoksch B, Ablassmaier B, Walter M, et al. Complication rate after thoracoscopic and conventional lobectomy. Zentralblatt fur Chirurgie 2003;128(2): 106–10.

[19] Giudicelli R, Thomas P, Lonjon T, et al. Major pulmonary resection by video assisted mini-thoracotomy. Initial experience in 35 patients. Eur J Cardiothorac Surg 1994;8:254–8.

[20] Walker WS. Video-assisted thoracic surgery (VATS) lobectomy: the Edinburgh experience. Semin Thorac Cardiovasc Surg 1998;10:291.

[21] Nakata M, Saeki H, Yokoyama N, et al. Pulmonary function after lobectomy: video-assisted thoracic surgery versus thoracotomy. Ann Thorac Surg 2000;70(3):938–41.

[22] Nomori H, Ohtsuka T, Horio H, et al. Difference in the impairment of vital capacity and 6-minute walking after a lobectomy performed by thoracoscopic surgery, an anterior limited thoracotomy, an antero-axillary thoracotomy, and a posterolateral thoracotomy. Surg Today 2003;33(1):7–12.

[23] Li WW, Lee RL, Lee TW, et al. The impact of thoracic surgical access on early shoulder function: video-assisted thoracic surgery versus posterolateral thoracotomy. Eur J Cardiothorac Surg 2003;23(3):390–6.

[24] Landreneau RJ, et al. Prevalence of chronic pain following pulmonary resection by thoracotomy or video-assisted thoracic surgery. J Thorac Cardiovasc Surg 1994;107:1079.

[25] Sugi K, Sudoh M, Hirazawa K, et al. Intrathoracic bleeding during video-assisted thoracoscopic lobectomy and segmentectomy. Jap J Thorac Surg 2003; 56(11):928–31.

[26] Kaseda S, Aoki T. Video-assisted thoracic surgical lobectomy in conjunction with lymphadenectomy for lung cancer. J Jap Surg Soc 2002;103(10): 717–21.

[27] Yim AP, Wan S, Lee TW, et al. VATS lobectomy reduces cytokine responses compared with conventional surgery. Ann Thorac Surg 2000;70(1):243–7.

[28] McKenna RJ Jr, Fischel RJ, Wolf R, et al. Is VATS lobectomy an adequate cancer operation? Ann Thorac Surg 1998;66:1903–8.

THORACIC
SURGERY
CLINICS

Thorac Surg Clin 17 (2007) 233–239

Variation in the Approach to VATS Lobectomy: Effect on the Evaluation of Surgical Morbidity Following VATS Lobectomy for the Treatment of Stage I Non–Small Cell Lung Cancer

Norihisa Shigemura, MD, PhD[a],
Anthony P.C. Yim, MD, FRCS, FACS[b],*

[a]*Division of Thoracic Surgery, The Heart, Lung, and Esophageal Surgery Institute, University of Pittsburgh Medical Center, Suite C800 PUH, 200 Lothrop Street, Pittsburgh, PA 15213, USA*
[b]*Division of Cardiothoracic Surgery, Department of Surgery, Chinese University of Hong Kong, Prince of Wales Hospital, Shatin, N.T., Hong Kong*

Recent advances in imaging, such as positron emission tomography, in chemical pathology, such as epidermal growth factor receptor expression and tumor markers, and in target therapy have made it necessary to redefine the role of surgery in the therapeutic algorithm in the management of lung cancer. Although video-assisted thoracic surgery (VATS) lobectomy with hilar and mediastinal lymph nodes dissection was proposed over a decade ago to treat early lung cancer, this technique is not widely practiced, despite many documented advantages (less postoperative pain, faster recovery, and better preserved pulmonary function and immune function). This article examines the role of VATS lobectomy in the treatment of early lung cancer and, in particular, the variations in the approach and the published results.

Video-assisted thoracic surgery major lung resection: a unified approach?

For over a decade, VATS has been embraced by the thoracic community as an acceptable, sometimes preferred approach to the management of a wide variety of thoracic conditions. Opinions regarding a VATS approach for major pulmonary resection (lobectomy or pneumonectomy) are divided, however, regarding its safety, oncologic clearance, long-term benefits, and cost effectiveness. An early, small, multi-institutional, randomized study of lobectomy failed to demonstrate any benefit of VATS over conventional thoracotomy [1]. One problem with this type of study, however, is that major resection by VATS is not a unified technique.

The techniques of VATS lobectomy vary greatly among institutions, and VATS lobectomy actually covers a broad spectrum of techniques that range from complete endoscopic surgery to minithoracotomy with a thoracoscope serving only as a light source [2]. Further, there is little consensus over some details of the technique. For example, how long an incision does one allow for minithoracotomy before it becomes a thoracotomy? How often should one operate through the minithoracotomy as opposed to the video monitor? How much rib spreading can be afforded before the benefits of minimal access surgery are lost? This variability in VATS techniques may contribute to confusion regarding the benefits of VATS lobectomy in the management of lung cancer. The authors believe that VATS lobectomy can be defined as a video-assisted, minimal-access technique in which the surgeon operates primarily by watching the television monitor, and little or no rib spreading is required throughout the entire procedure.

---

* Corresponding author.
 E-mail address: yimap@cuhk.edu.hk (A.P.C. Yim).

In addition, it should be realized that different VATS lobectomy techniques may yield different postoperative outcomes. The currently published, larger series on VATS major resections, which are believed to follow the previously mentioned definition of VATS lobectomy, are summarized in Table 1 [3–13], demonstrating that there are significant differences in operation time (79–246 minutes), morbidity rate (0.5%–21%), and mortality rate (0%–3.6%) even among the most experienced surgeons. A simple comparison of VATS lobectomy, as a group of many techniques, with other approaches that focus on a single aspect like mortality or major morbidity is neither proper nor meaningful, and the results may even be misleading [14].

Because inasmuch as major resection for early lung cancer (stage I) has become a common operation (one of the most common for a general thoracic surgeon), even a slight advantage of one technique over another could have far-reaching implications. Keeping this premise and facts in mind, it is imperative to develop a better assessment of this technique to stay with the scientific pursuit.

Assessment of the success of the approach

Quality of life

It is now fairly well established that patients who undergo VATS have less early postoperative pain compared with thoracotomy, by objective assessment of analgesic requirement or by subjective assessment of pain score [15,16]. In addition, one of the few prospective studies from the authors' unit has also shown that VATS can better preserve shoulder function compared with posterolateral thoracotomy [17]. Landreneau and colleagues [18] also found in their prospective, nonrandomized study with 138 patients that VATS was associated with significantly better short-term shoulder strength 3 weeks after surgery, although no significant differences were found between VATS and lateral thoracotomy more than 1 year after surgery. Postoperative shoulder dysfunction is an important factor in determining return to normal preoperative functioning and could become a serious long-term disability if neglected.

There have been very few reports on a study comparing the effects on the quality of life among many VATS techniques. Shigemura and colleagues [14] assessed the analgesic requirements

Table 1
Variations in video-assisted thoracic surgery lobectomy techniques

Author	Year	N	Minithoracotomy Position	Skin Incision (cm)	Rib-spreading	Direct or Monitor Vision	Operation Time (min)	% Morbidity	% Mortality
Kaseda et al [3]	1997	36	Anterolateral	8	No	100% monitor	295	n.c.	0
Iwasaki et al [4]	1998	100	Anterior and posterior (two-windows)	3 (window)	n.c.	n.c.	166	n.c.	n.c.
Lewis et al [5]	2000	85	Lateral	5	No	100% monitor	79	13	0
Naruke et al [23]	2000	60	Middle axillary	7	No	n.c.	n.c.	n.c.	0
Yim [7]	2002	266	Anterolateral	6	No	100% monitor	90	0.50	0
Walker et al [8,24]	2002	158	Anterolateral	5	n.c.	n.c.	130	n.c.	1.80
Daniels et al [9]	2002	90	Anterior	4.5	No	100% monitor	n.c.	19.10	3.60
Gharagozloo et al [10]	2003	179	Not used (3-port only)	2 (port)	No	100% monitor	n.c.	21	0.05
Roviaro et al [11]	2004	193	Inframammary	4	No	100% monitor	n.c.	n.c.	1.03
McKenna et al [12]	2006	966	Lateral	4	No	100% monitor	n.c.	15.30	0.80
Shigemura et al [13]	2006	56	Middle axillary	4	No	100% monitor	246	6	0

Abbreviation: n.c., not commented in the original.

together with postoperative serum inflammatory markers between complete VATS without and assisted VATS with the use of rib-spreader for utility thoracotomy. They found that although there was no significant difference in analgesic use, serum peak levels of postoperative inflammatory markers (white blood cell counts, C-reactive protein, creatine phosphokinase) were lower with complete VATS and earlier return to normalization than with assisted VATS, which may translate into an improved quality-of-life with faster recovery from the surgery for patients. Although more proper comparative studies using standardized questionnaires and objective evaluations regarding quality-of-life assessments should be done, one can emphasize that the advantages associated with the true VATS lobectomy techniques are attributable to the avoidance of rib spreading, and the use of VATS assistance during minithoracotomy with a rib-spreader does not confer these advantages.

Further, in the past several years, there have been tremendous advancements in the field of adjuvant chemotherapy for patients with lung cancer [19], and this therapeutic modality is expected to play an increasing role in lung cancer management. Because chemotherapy produces superior outcomes in patients with better functional status reflected in quality of life, the use of surgical techniques that preserve functional status from the least traumatic VATS techniques may allow earlier commencement of adjuvant chemotherapy and may lead to better outcomes.

Lymph node dissection

Lymph node dissection in lung cancer surgery continues to be a subject of considerable controversy. The debate relates not so much to the type of surgical approach used but to the desirability in performing lymphadenectomy in patients with early lung cancer. The protagonists, including many leading Japanese surgeons, agree that lymphadenectomy can be performed with little added morbidity, and can more accurately stage patients, so it should be routinely performed [20,21]. The antagonists, however, agree that there are no proved therapeutic benefits in lymphadenectomy, and systematic lymph node sampling provides an alternative in surgical staging. The whole issue is currently the subject of a major rational randomized trial under the American College of Surgeons Oncology Group. Irrespective of the outcome, however, it must be realized

that medical imaging has advanced significantly over the past years. Positron emission tomography and other imaging modalities on the horizon promise to impact significantly on the way surgeons deal with the mediastinum.

Suffice for now, however, the technical feasibility of a complete lymphadenectomy through the VATS approach is examined. Among a variety of many VATS lobectomy techniques, there have been few published reports on whether or not there is difference in the quality of lymph node dissection. Sagawa and colleagues [22], in a prospective trial of systematic nodal dissection by VATS, reported that they missed few lymph nodes with VATS as compared with conventional open thoracotomy. The latest report by Shigemura and colleagues [13] also demonstrated statistically that there is no difference in the quality of a complete dissection by enumerating the lymph nodes removed between complete VATS and assisted VATS approaches and the open conventional approach. They found that the number of dissected lymph nodes by complete VATS (23 ± 9) was equivalent to those by assisted VATS (22 ± 6; $P =$ not significant) and the conventional approach (25 ± 7; $P =$ not significant), whereas the long-term survival benefits were also equivalent.

Also considered is that there are patients in whom lymph node dissection is not indicated as other authors suggested (eg, those who have in situ bronchioalveolar cell carcinoma or squamous cell cancer ≤ 2 cm in diameter, in whom nodal metastases rarely occur). Naruke and colleagues [23], based on the meticulous analysis of 1815 patients who underwent systematic lymph node dissection and complete resection, previously advocated that sentinel lymph node sampling might provide an alternative strategy for surgeons to decide on the necessity of complete mediastinal node dissection for those cases of clinical T1N0 small-sized lung cancer. Systematic sampling of the sentinel lymph node in ensuring the N staging using minimally invasive technique, followed by determining the need for complete lymph node dissection, may be a convincing option with more evidence established.

The authors believe that systematic lymph node investigation, regardless of either dissection or sampling, is routinely indicated for stage I lung cancer to yield accurate staging. Based on this principle, when judging the success of one VATS lobectomy technique as lung cancer operation, the quality of lymph node investigation may play a pivotal role together with the long-term survival benefits.

Long-term survival

The success of a cancer operation is judged ultimately by the long-term survival of the treated patients. Several centers have reported their extensive experience and follow-up. Naruke [6] reported his excellent survival after VATS lobectomy for pathologic T1N0M0 was 100% at 4 years; Yim [7], 95% at 26 months; and Gharagozloo and colleagues [10] 85% at 5 years. Shigemura and associates [13] recently demonstrated that their 5-year survival of patients with peripheral lung cancer less than or equal to 2 cm in diameter (stage IA) was 96.7% following complete VATS, 95.2% following minithoracotomy with video assistance, and 97.2% following open surgery, revealing that long-term survival was comparable among different VATS lobectomy techniques and conventional method (Table 2) [1–11]. Confirmation of the oncologic effectiveness of VATS lobectomy is best demonstrated by a large, prospective, randomized,

controlled series. Most thoracic surgeons, however, especially VATS surgeons, realize that it is not forthcoming because of the lack of convincing reasons to permit randomization.

There is now a growing evidence to suggest that the body's immune function is better preserved following VATS compared with thoracotomy as documented by release of proinflammatory and anti-inflammatory cytokines, circulating T cells (CD4) and natural killer (NK) cells, and lymphocyte oxidation [24–26]. Because immunosurveillance is believed to be important, surgically induced immunosuppression may predispose to increased tumor growth and recurrence. Whether or not better preservation of the immune function through minimization of chest wall trauma by VATS is the explanation behind the observed improved intermediate- to long-term survival is unclear, but the authors believe this certainly deserves further investigation. Besides the clinical outcomes including the long-term survival data,

Table 2
Assessment of the success of the approach in video-assisted thoracic surgery lobectomy for lung cancer

Author	Year	How to assess the quality of life	Lymph node (LN) dissection (D)/sampling (S)	How to assess the quality of LN dissection	Long-term (follow-up)
Kaseda et al [3]	1997	n.c.	Systematic D with details	Number of resected nodes	No recurrence (median 17 mo)
Iwasaki et al [4]	1998	Pulmonary function test at 1 month	Systematic D with details	Number of resected nodes	n.c.
Lewis et al [5]	2000	Time for return to work	Systematic D with details	n.c.	n.c.
Naruke et al [23]	2000	n.c.	Systematic D with details	According to map as a guide	100% (60 mo)
Yim [7]	2002	Cytokine (inerleukin-6), shoulder function	Systematic S	n.c.	95% (26 mo)
Walker et al [8,24]	2002	Cytokine, white cell function	Systematic S	n.c.	77% (60 mo)
Daniels et al [9]	2002	n.c.	Systematic D with details	n.c.	n.c.
Gharagozloo et al [10]	2003	n.c.	Systematic S	n.c.	85% (60 mo)
Roviaro et al [11]	2004	n.c.	Systematic S	n.c.	70% (60 mo)
McKenna et al [12]	2006	n.c.	Systematic D with details	n.c.	75% (60 mo)
Shigemura et al [13]	2006	Inflammatory marker (WBC, CRP, CPK)	Systematic D with details	Number of resected nodes for comparison	96% (60 mo)

Abbreviations: CPK, creatine phosphokinase; CRP, C-reactive protein; n.c., not commented in the original; WBC, white blood cell counts.

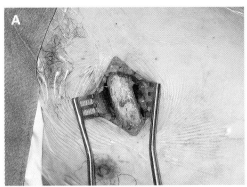

Fig. 1. Segmental rib resection method number 1. Minithoracotomy with a segment of the underlying rib explored (*A*), and after rib resection to reveal the underlying lung (*B*). Only a soft tissue retractor was used throughout. (*From* Shigemura N, Hsin MK, Yim APC. Segmental rib resection for difficult cases of video-assisted thoracic surgery. J Thorac Cardiovasc Surg 2006;132:701–2; with permission.)

one should consider accumulating the series of evidence behind the superiority of VATS approach over the conventional way, such as this kind of basic research data, which are scientifically convincing enough for all doctors, regardless of their specialties.

Segmental rib resection in video-assisted thoracic surgery: a new direction?

Although several variations exist in VATS techniques, recently the authors also reported a strategy that adds a new dimension to this spectrum of techniques [27]. By resecting a segment of rib underneath the utility minithoracotomy, without rib spreading, the surgeon can perform difficult VATS cases safely and easily with conventional thoracic instruments (Figs. 1 and 2). The authors have used this approach in their institution for more than 150 consecutive cases of difficult VATS major resections without complications. These include redo VATS, stage 3A lung cancer after neoadjuvant chemotherapy, and for parenchymal lung tumors larger than 3 cm. Postoperative pain among patients who underwent VATS with rib resection does not seem to differ from that of patients who did not have rib resection in terms of analgesic requirements. They have recently applied this approach for patients with stage I lung cancer, especially in cases when the chief thoracic residents attempt VATS lobectomy.

When one considers that one of the reasons the application of VATS to major pulmonary resections is still not widely practiced is that many surgeons may still perceive this operation to be

technically demanding, rib resection method would be useful to experienced VATS surgeons dealing with difficult cases and to beginner VATS surgeons learning complex VATS procedures. The authors believe this approach may lead to wider acceptance of VATS major pulmonary resection in the thoracic surgical community.

Video-assisted thoracic surgery lobectomy as a lung cancer operation

Initially viewed as a heresy, VATS lobectomy has matured to become an established, alternative approach to conventional open surgery for patients with early stage lung cancer. It is a safe

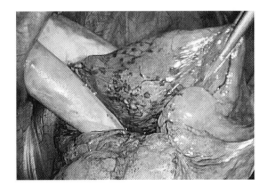

Fig. 2. Segmental rib resection method number 2. Bidigital palpation of the specimen can be easily performed through the minithoracotomy, in this case to identify a deeply seated lung nodule. (*From* Shigemura N, Hsin MK, Yim APC. Segmental rib resection for difficult cases of video-assisted thoracic surgery. J Thorac Cardiovasc Surg 2006;132:701–2; with permission.)

procedure in experienced hands, and more recent studies suggest that benefits may go well beyond the early postoperative period to intermediate- to long-term survival, especially with stage I lung cancer. As the documented benefits of VATS resection start to accumulate, it will be increasingly difficult to justify not using VATS as the surgical approach of choice in selected patients.

Although VATS lobectomy has not achieved the expected widespread acceptance seen with other minimally invasive procedures, the authors believe that the recent outstanding advancements in the field of adjuvant chemotherapy for patients with lung cancer should force the focus again on the proved advantages of this evolving approach. Because chemotherapy produces better outcomes in patients with better functional status, oncologists expect a minimally invasive but complete cancer operation. If clinicians can provide both of the benefits to patients in a strict sense, it will be possible to recruit patients, and ultimately improve their survival in cooperation with physicians.

Variation in techniques for an evolving procedure is understandable; however, a distinction in these operative techniques together with scientifically proved, convincing assessment of them must be made before a meaningful comparison of results can be made. Further, one must keep in mind that the term "VATS lobectomy" should be reserved to the predominantly endoscopic technique with no rib spreading, which has been shown to provide benefits recognized in minimally invasive surgery.

References

[1] Kirby TJ, Mack MJ, Landreneau RJ, et al. Lobectomy-video assisted thoracic surgery versus muscle-sparing thoracotomy: a randomized trial. J Thorac Cardiovasc Surg 1995;109:997–1002.

[2] Yim AP, Landreneau RJ, Izzat MB, et al. Is video-assisted thoracoscopic lobectomy a unified approach? Ann Thorac Surg 1998;66:1155–8.

[3] Kaseda S, Hangai N, Yamamoto S, et al. Lobectomy with extended lymph node dissection by video-assisted thoracic surgery for lung cancer. Surg Endosc 1997;11:703–6.

[4] Iwasaki M, Kaga K, Nishiumi N, et al. Experience with the two-windows method for mediastinal lymph node dissection in lung cancer. Ann Thorac Surg 1998;65:800–2.

[5] Lewis RJ, Caccavale RJ, Boncage JP, et al. Video-assisted thoracic surgical non-rib spreading simultaneously stapled lobectomy: a more patient-friendly oncologic resection. Chest 1999;116:1119–24.

[6] Naruke T. Thoracoscopic lobectomy with mediastinal lymph node dissection or sampling. In: Yim AP, editor. Minimal access cardiothoracic surgery. Philadelphia: WB Saunders; 2000. p. 110–24.

[7] Yim AP. VATS major pulmonary resection revisited: controversies, techniques, and results. Ann Thorac Surg 2002;74:615–23.

[8] Walker WS, Codispoti M, Soon SY, et al. Long-term outcomes following VATS lobectomy for non-small cell bronchogenic carcinoma. Eur J Cardiothorac Surg 2001;20:455–63.

[9] Daniels LJ, Balderson SS, Onaitis MW, et al. Thoracoscopic lobectomy: a safe and effective strategy for patients with stage I lung cancer. Ann Thorac Surg 2002;74:860–4.

[10] Gharagozloo F, Tempesta B, Margolis M, et al. Video-assisted thoracoscopic surgery lobectomy for stage I lung cancer. Ann Thorac Surg 2003;76: 1009–15.

[11] Roviaro G, Varoli F, Vergani C, et al. Long-term survival after videothoracoscopic lobectomy for stage I lung cancer. Chest 2004;126:725–32.

[12] McKenna RJ, Houck W, Fuller CB. Video-assisted thoracic surgery lobectomy: experience with 1000 cases. Ann Thorac Surg 2006;81:421–6.

[13] Shigemura N, Akashi A, Funaki S, et al. Long-term outcomes after a variety of video-assisted thoracoscopic lobectomy approaches for clinical stage IA lung cancer: a multi-institutional study. J Thorac Cardiovasc Surg 2006;132:507–12.

[14] Shigemura N, Akashi A, Nakagiri T, et al. Complete vs assisted thoracoscopic approach: a prospective randomized trial comparing a variety of video-assisted thoracoscopic lobectomy techniques. Surg Endosc 2004;18:1492–7.

[15] Landreneau RJ, Hazelrigg SR, Mack MJ, et al. Postoperative pain-related morbidity: video-assisted thoracic surgery versus thoracotomy. Ann Thorac Surg 1993;56:1285–9.

[16] Yim AP. Minimizing chest wall trauma in video-assisted thoracic surgery. J Thorac Cardiovasc Surg 1995;109:1255–6.

[17] Li WW, Lee RL, Lee TW, et al. The impact of thoracic surgical access on early shoulder function: video-assisted thoracic surgery versus posterolateral thoracotomy. Eur J Cardiothorac Surg 2003;23: 390–6.

[18] Landreneau RJ, Mack MJ, Hazelrigg SR, et al. Prevalence of chronic pain after pulmonary resection by thoracotomy or video-assisted thoracic surgery. J Thorac Cardiovasc Surg 1994;107:1079–86.

[19] Winton TL, Livingston R, Johnson D, et al. Vinorelbine plus cisplatin vs. observation in resected non-small cell lung cancer. N Engl J Med 2005;352: 2589–97.

[20] Naruke T, Suemasu K, Ishikawa S. Lymph node mapping and curability at various levels of metastasis in resected lung cancer. J Thorac Cardiovasc Surg 1978;76:832–9.

[21] Asamura H, Nakayama H, Kondo H, et al. Lymph node metastases, recurrence, and prognosis in resected small, peripheral, non-small-cell lung carcinomas: are these carcinomas candidates for video-assisted lobectomy? J Thorac Cardiovasc Surg 1996;110:1125–34.

[22] Sagawa M, Sato M, Sakurada A, et al. A prospective trial of systematic nodal dissection for lung cancer by video-assisted thoracic surgery: can it be perfect? Ann Thorac Surg 2002;73:900–4.

[23] Naruke T, Tsuchiya R, Kondo H, et al. Lymph node sampling in lung cancer: how should it be done? Eur J Cardiothorac Surg 1999;16:S17–24.

[24] Walker WS. The immune response to surgery: conventional and VATS lobectomy. In: Yim AP, Hazelrigg SR, Izzat MB, et al, editors. Minimal access cardiothoracic surgery. Philadelphia: WB Saunders; 2000. p. 127–34.

[25] Yim AP, Wan S, Lee TW, et al. VATS lobectomy reduces cytokine responses compared with conventional surgery. Ann Thorac Surg 2000;70:243–7.

[26] Ng CS, Whealan RL, Lacy AM, et al. Is minimal access surgery for cancer associated with immunologic benefits? World J Surg 2005;29:975–81.

[27] Shigemura N, Hsin M, Yim APC. Segmental rib resection for difficult video-assisted cases. J Thorac Cardiovasc Surg 2006;132:701–2.

THORACIC
SURGERY
CLINICS

Thorac Surg Clin 17 (2007) 241–249

Immunologic and Stress Responses Following Video-Assisted Thoracic Surgery and Open Pulmonary Lobectomy in Early Stage Lung Cancer

William S. Walker, FRCS[a],*, H. Anne Leaver, PhD[b]

[a]Department of Thoracic Surgery, Royal Infirmary of Edinburgh, Little France, Edinburgh, EH16 4SA, Scotland, UK
[b]Cell Biology Laboratory, Blood Transfusion R&D, Scottish National Blood Transfusion Service, Edinburgh, EH17 7QT, Scotland, UK

Surgery in whatever form constitutes an injury process. Consequent upon this, a variety of physiologic and immunologic stress responses is generated. Over centuries, various strategies have evolved that attempt to minimize the effect of surgical interventions. These have included surgical speed, optimizing pain relief, antisepsis and antibiotic therapy, technical delicacy and precision, and, recently, minimal access approaches. The relationship between stress responses and cancer is a matter of crucial interest for thoracic surgeons, because there is evidence that disturbances associated with the stress response may reduce resistance to the growth and spread of cancer, due in part to impairment of cellular immune mechanisms. This article considers the nature of the injury responses, assesses the degree to which they may be modified by a minimal access strategy, and draws together the potential implications of these investigations for the surgical management of early-stage lung cancer.

The stress response

Multiple inputs contribute to and modify the surgical response to injury (Fig. 1). This process may be considered as having endocrine, neural, and immunologic components [1], all of which are subject to varying degrees of mutual interaction (Box 1).

___

* Corresponding author.
E-mail address: wsw@holyrood.ed.ac.uk
(W.S. Walker).

The evolution of our understanding of the stress response to surgery has been reviewed in detail elsewhere [2], and the general metabolic response to surgery is summarized in Table 1. The importance of neural afferent stimuli in the generation of the stress response, although less immediately obvious to the surgeon than the degree of tissue trauma, has been confirmed in experimental and clinical studies that demonstrated that epidural anesthesia reduces stress responses, improves perioperative mortality, and reduces postsurgical morbidity [3]. Neural effector mechanisms in the stress response include direct hypothalamic stimulation, epinephrine release from the adrenal medulla, diffusion of norepinephrine from presynaptic nerve terminals, rennin secretion by the juxtaglomerular apparatus, and hypothalamic stimulation.

Tissue trauma generates a wide range of immunologic responses (Fig. 2). Cytokines, chemokines, growth factors, lipids [4,5], and other mediators are released by activated leucocytes, macrophages, fibroblasts, and endothelial cells and are involved in the local injury response and in the systemic reaction. Although there are parallel and interacting processes involved, from a surgical perspective, a major initiating process involves the activation and recruitment of macrophages and monocytes by tissue damage leading to release of interleukin (IL)-1 and tumor necrosis factor α (TNF-α), which cause the release of IL-6. These cytokines are those most studied in the surgical literature.

IL-1 and TNF have been implicated in the immune response to surgery. IL-1, derived from

Physiological Responses to Surgery - Origins

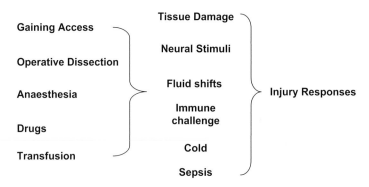

Fig. 1. Physiologic responses to surgery: origins.

pro–IL-1 by the action of caspase-1, signals the activation of proinflammatory enzymes and has profound effects on the endothelium involving prostaglandin E_2 (PGE_2) [4,5], inducible nitric oxide synthetase, and intercellular adhesion molecules. TNF-α, the major cytokine secreted by activated macrophages, regulates apoptosis and depresses myocardial function. IL-6 production, which is induced by TNF-α and IL-1β (whose production IL-6 suppresses as an anti-inflammatory effect), also has been implicated in cellular stress responses. Thus, levels of IL-6 are proportionate to injury, and this cytokine is the most commonly used quantitative marker in surgical studies. IL-6 generates pyrexia, activates the hypothalamic pituitary axis, and dictates the hepatic acute-phase protein response (C-reactive protein [CRP], fibrinogen, α2macroglobulin, antiproteinases) and transport proteins. Glucocorticoids produce negative feedback on IL-6 secretion. The effects of these and other surgically relevant cytokines have been well summarized by Raeburn and colleagues [6]. There are, however, 30 such proteins, many of which have important immunoregulatory functions. The predominant immunologic effects of major surgery are presented in Table 2.

Although the main area of interest in this article is the nature of immunologic and cytokine responses in open and video-assisted thoracic surgery (VATS) major pulmonary resection, it is important to appreciate that these changes do not exist in isolation, but rather as part of the broad range of physiologic mechanisms associated with injury.

Relationship between immune mechanisms and cancer

Patients who have lung cancer undergo major stress against a background of preexisting compromise. For example, CD4, CD8, and natural killer (NK) cell numbers are already suppressed in this group [7]. Therefore, it is relevant to briefly consider the current thinking with regard to immune mechanisms and cancer. This is well reviewed elsewhere [8–11].

Box 1. Physiologic responses to surgery

Endocrine response
Pituitary hormone secretion
Insulin resistance

Sympathetic nervous system stimulation
Catecholamine release
Tachycardia and hypertension
Modified hepatic, pancreatic, pulmonary, and renal function

Immunologic changes
Cytokine and local mediator production
Acute-phase and stress pathway reactions
Neutrophil leukocytosis and secretion
Lymphocytic proliferation and activation

———
Data from Desborough JP. The stress response to trauma and surgery. Br J Anaesth 2000;85(1):109–17.

Table 1
Summary of metabolic response to surgery

Carbohydrate	Hyperglycemia	Hepatic glycogenolysis and gluconeogenesis
		Decreased peripheral use
		Insulin resistance
Protein	Catabolism	Skeletal muscle breakdown
		Amino acids used for gluconeogenesis or
		Manufacture of acute phase proteins
Fat	Breakdown	Glycerol → gluconeogenesis
		FFAs → ketones/oxidation/re-esterified
Fluid and electrolyte	Water retention	ADH effect lasts 3–5 days
	Na retention	Renin/aldosterone → Na retention
	Changes in divalent ions	↑Cu++, ↓ Zn++, ↓ Fe++; reflects carrier protein metabolism

Adaptive immunity (ie, that related to antibody production) has limited relevance because tumors generally (and lung cancer, in particular) are of low antigenicity. Also, patients with immunodeficiencies (as opposed to immunosuppression) do not experience a marked increase in solid tumor development. Innate immunity, however, may play a significant role in the control and suppression of malignancy by way of macrophage, T-cell, and NK cell actions. Macrophages can infiltrate a tumor mass in vitro and destroy cells by way of production of reactive oxygen intermediate (ROI) species and TNF when activated by various factors, including T-cell gamma interferon (IFNγ). It is believed that tumor antigenic fragments are recognized by dendritic cells (DCs) and transported to local lymph nodes where they are presented by the DCs to T cells that are then stimulated to attack the tumor cells (Fig. 3).

Generally, NK cells are considered to provide a primary cellular effector mechanism against dissemination of blood-borne metastases and exhibit decreased levels in advanced metastatic disease. Resting NK cells are spontaneously cytolytic for certain malignant cell types and following IL-2 activation, NK cells acquire a wider target range. Liver-associated NK cells have higher expression of IL-2 receptor and adhesion molecules than do circulating NK cells. Liver-associated NK cells are precursors of activated adherent NK cells. These adhere rapidly to solid surfaces under the influence of IL-2 and are more effective at entering solid tumors. Nonadherent NK cells show selective cytotoxicity against

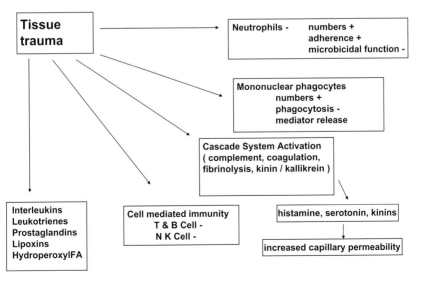

Fig. 2. Immunologic responses to tissue trauma.

Table 2
Predominant immunologic effects of major surgery

Decreased	IL-2 production
	IL-2 receptor expression
	IFN-γ production
Decreased	T-cell blastogenesis and number
	NK cell activity
	LAK cell activity
Increased	Fas-mediated apoptosis of
	circulating lymphocytes
Adverse	T-cell subpopulation changes:
	$\downarrow$CD4, $\uparrow$ or $\rightarrow$ CD8
Impaired	Monocyte and neutrophil function
	Chemoattractance $\downarrow$
	Phagocytosis $\downarrow$
	O_2 free radical release $\uparrow$
	$\uparrow$ Phagocyte PGE$_2$ secretion

Abbreviations: LAK, lymphokine activated killer cell; $\uparrow$, increased; $\downarrow$, decreased; $\rightarrow$, unchanged.
Data from Kehlet, 1998; Leaver, 2000.

antibody-coated cancer cells through antibody-dependent cellular cytotoxicity. Therefore, the effects of minimally invasive surgery on specific NK cell subpopulations (and, if possible also on linked tumor explants) and lung tumor antigens

should be considered in addition to total NK population dynamic studies [10,12].

Tumor escape mechanisms

The various mechanisms involving innate and adaptive immunologic systems by which tumors may avoid immune recognition are summarized in Table 3. The process whereby tumors flourish, despite host immune mechanisms, is described by two models: the immunosurveillance and danger models. The surveillance model proposes a process of "cancer immunoediting," by which strongly immunogenic tumors are selected out early and less immunogenic cells subsequently escape immunosurveillance. The danger model concentrates on the recognition of danger signals by antigen-processing cells (DCs, macrophages, and B cells), which stimulate T-cell responses. Defective antigen presentation is more common in metastases than in primary tumors, and there is evidence that tumors may escape immunosurveillance by several routes.

Cell-mediated and innate immune responses are believed to play an important role in lung cancer pathophysiology. It is believed that T cells,

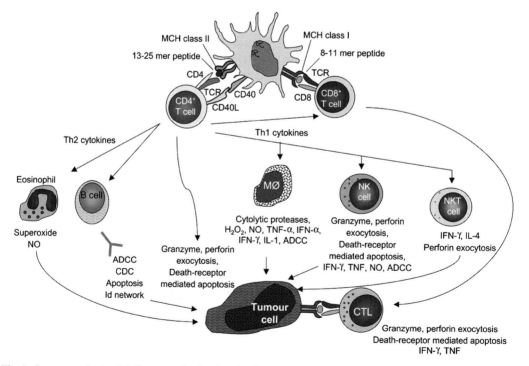

Fig. 3. Summary of potential effector mechanism involved in antitumour immunity. ADCC, antibody dependent cellular toxicity; CDC, complement dependent cytotoxicity; CTL, cytotoxic T cell; TCR, T cell receptor. (*From* Mosolits S, Ullenhag G, Mellstedt H. Therapeutic vaccination in patients with gastrointestinal malignancies. A review of immunological and clinical results. Ann Oncol 2005;16:847–62; with permission from the European Society for Medical Oncology.)

Table 3
Tumor escape mechanisms

Mechanism	Result
Down-regulation of HLA class I molecules	Tumor cells less attractive to cytotoxic T cells
Impaired antigen presentation	Tumors may create a microenvironment that results in imbalances in antigen-presenting cell (APC) subsets (eg, DCs) that fail to express appropriate costimulatory molecules. APCs that deliver antigen in the absence of CD28 ligands render T cells anergic. This "active tolerance"process may be due to loss of signals that up-regulate costimulatory molecules on APCs.
Growth\angiogenic factors	Factors, such as vascular endothelial growth factor (VEGF), are secreted commonly by solid tumors and promote growth of new blood vessels. VEGF also suppresses DC activity.
Surface molecule expression	FasL and a growth inhibitory molecule RCAS1 that increase T-cell apoptosis and down-regulation of tumor adhesion and activation molecules
Cytokine and immunosuppressive factors	Tumors may secrete TGFβ and IL-10, which exert an immunosuppressive effect by way of PGE_2 and may provide local protection, even when large numbers of tumor-specific CD8 cells are present in peripheral blood
Immunogenomic/epigenetic factors	DNA methylation of immune genes, oncogenes, and environmental mutagenic stimuliHistone acetylation, MAP kinase signaling

Abbreviations: HLA, human leukocyte antigen; MAP, mitogen-activated protein; TGF, transforming growth factor.

rather than antibodies, attack solid tumors, particularly those expressing intracellular antigens on their surface. Because most of these are major histocompatibility complex class II negative, it is likely that CD8 (cytotoxic) T-cell responses play an important role. CD4 (helper) T cells also are involved in protective mechanisms against tumor-associated vasculature and are required for persistence of CD8 T cells. Local immunomodulatory factors, such as growth factors, cell surface molecules, local cytokines, and mediators, form a microenvironment that determines immune cell and tumor gene function [1,4,6,9,13–15]. For example, PGE_2 has potent immunoinhibitory activity with respect to monocyte, T-cell, and NK cell action and may influence tumor proliferation and metastasis [4,5,15]. Environmental factors also play specific roles in the molecular pathways of lung cancer development, in which, for example, inflammatory mediators and tissue DNA methylation may be linked with smoking [10].

Comparison of video-assisted thoracic surgery and open lobectomy

Endocrine and neuroendocrine responses

Endocrine and sympathetic nervous system responses to surgery have been studied in some

detail in relation to a wide range of laparoscopic procedures, including cholecystectomy, herniorrhaphy, colonic resection, hysterectomy, and various other procedures and reviewed in detail by Kehlet [13]. Typically, corticotropin, cortisol, prolactin, and catecholamines were studied. In general, there is little evidence for a significant difference in endocrine responses between open and laparoscopic procedures; however, only one endocrine study comparing VATS with open surgery has been performed [16]. This study compared VATS wedge with a transaxillary thoracotomy approach and noted reduced epinephrine levels in the group that underwent VATS, but similar norepinephrine levels in both groups.

Immunologic and stress cytokine studies

In contrast to endocrine studies, investigators comparing laparoscopic or VATS approaches with open surgery have noted significant differences between minimally invasive and open approaches. Laparoscopic surgery outcomes were reviewed in detail by Kehlet [13]. Laparoscopy is associated commonly with less generation of IL-6 and CRP. Also, leucocytosis is reduced. A reduction in the shift in the type 1/type 2 T helper–cell balance toward type 2 cells was noted by Decker and colleagues [17], who compared laparoscopic and open cholecystectomy implying less down-regulation of cell-mediated immunity. Reduced dysregulation of T-cell function has been described using the same model [18]. Better preservation of lymphocyte numbers [19] and quicker return of lymphocyte proliferative responses to normal also have been reported with laparoscopic colon resection [20].

Few immunologic studies have been reported for VATS cases. Gebhardt [21] compared open and VATS surgery for pneumothorax and found that CRP, thromboxane, and prostacyclin levels were lower in the group that underwent VATS. Most of the studies in this area have concentrated on comparisons between open and VATS lobectomy [12,22–26] and are summarized in Table 4. There are differences in approach between various VATS lobectomy techniques, but IL-6 and CRP reductions were demonstrated in several different studies [23–25]. Our experience [12,24] is based on a prospective randomized study of 41 patients undergoing lobectomy. We found significant differences in acute-phase and cellular immune responses between the two groups. We also noted that the VATS and open postoperative IL-6 profiles exhibited temporal differences, in addition to the reduced magnitude of IL-6 production associated with the VATS approach. IL-6 levels peaked within a few hours following VATS lobectomy, as compared with open lobectomy, when the peak occurred at about 24 hours (Fig. 4). Although this may partly reflect differences in incisional trauma, we believe that it also could reflect important differences in intraoperative lung trauma, because the lung is a major generator of cytokines and local mediators. Consistent with this hypothesis, Sugi and colleagues [22] reported that IL-6 levels in pleural fluid samples following lobectomy were more than 100 times higher than corresponding systemic levels. They also noted that the increase in IL-6 in pleural fluid 3 hours after surgery was significantly lower following VATS lobectomy compared with open lobectomy.

As with several laparoscopic studies, we [12,24] found that lymphocyte counts decreased after surgery but that VATS lobectomy was associated with less effect on circulating T (CD4) cells and on NK lymphocytes after surgery. Lymphocyte oxidation was less suppressed in the group that underwent VATS, and phagocyte generation of ROI species was less marked. Generation of ROI species is a specialized function of phagocytic cell types and an effector cell function in the cellular immune response. Basal oxidative activity may signal cell growth. Both functions affect circulating leucocytes in the perioperative period in patients with malignancy. The phagocytic oxidative response is relevant to tumor cell killing, whereas the proliferative response of leucocyte populations directs selective immune responses to specific epitopes and cytokine/mediator signals.

Discussion

The studies available for comparison between open and minimal access surgery have important

Table 4
Studies comparing immunologic and acute-phase responses in open and video-assisted thoracic surgery

Study	Comparison	Outcome with VATS compared to open
Leaver et al, 2000 [12]	VATS versus open lobectomy	↓ reduction in T (CD4) & NK (CD56,CD16) lymphocytes↓ suppression of lymphocytic oxidative activity
Yim et al, 2000 [23]	VATS versus open lobectomy	↓ generation of IL-6, -8, & -10
Sugi et al, 2000 [22,29]	VATS versus open lobectomy	IL-6, -8 in blood → ↓ generation of IL-6 in pleural fluid
Craig et al, 2001 [24]	VATS versus open lobectomy	↓ generation of CRP, IL-6↓ neutrophil & macrophage ROS surge
Nagahiro et al, 2001 [25]	VATS versus open lobectomy	↓ generation of IL-6
Kuda et al, 2002 [26]	VATS versus VATS with minithoracotomy	CRP, IL-6, WBC →
	Exploratory thoracotomy versus lobectomy	WBC count response less with exploratory thoracotomy

Abbreviations: ROS, reactive oxygen species; WBC, white blood cell; ↓, decreased; →, unchanged.

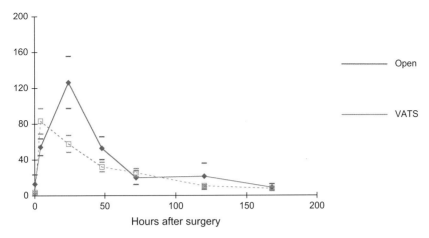

Fig. 4. IL-6 levels following open and VATS lobectomy.

limitations. As in many areas, we may be "measuring the measurable rather than the meaningful." Tissue active cytokines and other immunomodulatory factors may exhibit localized plasma and tissue levels. Sampling times are, of necessity, fixed, and therefore, may miss effects. Also, much of the area of greatest interest (ie, local immune mechanisms) involves interactions within microsystems (eg, the microenvironment of systemic and local mediators, cell–cell interactions, and cellular and tissue dynamics [migration, activation, signaling]). Furthermore, immunomodulatory signals are influenced by various factors, including specific circulating binding proteins, receptor variables and the effects of other cytokines, mediators, and cellular and secretory metabolism. Consequently, plasma levels of individual circulating cytokines may have limited significance. Furthermore, from a methodological perspective, the studies discussed above involve modest numbers of patients, multiple testing, and frequently are nonrandomized. It is unlikely that it will be possible to repeat these studies; for centers with active VATS programs, patients frequently are referred with the expectation of undergoing VATS resection.

Despite these formidable caveats, the available evidence suggests that although a minimally invasive approach has little effect on endocrine responses, laparoscopic and thoracoscopic studies show reduced acute-phase responses compared with open procedures and better preservation of cellular immune mechanisms. These studies indicate that targeting specific immunologic and stress response pathways may result in novel strategies to attenuate tumor development. Reducing surgical trauma as provided by a VATS approach offers one option. Other approaches include pharmacologic and gene therapy involving blockade of growth factors, their receptors, and inhibition of stress response cellular signaling mediators, including Ras, metalloprotease, and cyclooxygenase-2 [15].

Anesthesia and blood transfusion have potent negative effects on immune mechanisms [27,28], whereas in the experience of most surgeons, VATS lobectomy involves minimal stimulation and blood loss.

At the outset of VATS surgery, the focus was on the prospect for reducing pain and operative trauma with consequent reduction in hospitalization times and more rapid recovery to normal activity. These remain important objectives, and the argument in favor of VATS has largely been won for many nononcological procedures; however, uptake of VATS lobectomy remains remarkably low. The concern over cancer-related issues is an important driver for conservatism in this area. Conversely, review of published series demonstrates excellent survival data with VATS lobectomy for early-stage non-small cell lung cancer [29–33]. Although it is possible that a degree of selection bias may apply to the VATS cases, it seems that survival in stage I cases may be superior to that achieved using conventional techniques. Given that there may be a degree of understaging in the group that undergoes VATS because of less radical lymph node sampling/dissection, this effect is all the more striking.

Even for stage I cases, recurrence, when it occurs, is systemic in approximately 60% of cases. This implies tumor dissemination during surgery or the presence of micrometastatic disease at the time of resection. It is almost impossible to handle or squeeze the lung during minimally invasive surgery, as demonstrated by the reduced pleural fluid cytokine levels in VATS cases, suggesting that the risk for intraoperative dissemination should be reduced with this technique. With regard to micrometastases, it is tempting to speculate that the reduced trauma and pain associated with VATS lobectomy and consequent better preservation of immune mechanisms will provide a superior immunologic milieu in which to allow host defenses to operate more effectively. Immunotherapy is a major area of current research seeking to boost host defense and immune surveillance mechanisms [9,10,34,35].

Less traumatic surgery may offer a simple strategy to improve immune function further in the perioperative period.

Acknowledgments

We are grateful to Dr. Dino Rotondo (Strathclyde University, Glasgow, UK) and Dr. Maria Teresa Rizzo (Signal Transduction Laboratory, Indianapolis, Indiana) for critical analysis of the manuscript.

References

[1] Desborough JP. The stress response to trauma and surgery. Br J Anaesth 2000;85(1):109–17.

[2] Wilmore DW. From Cuthbertson to fast-track surgery: 70 years of progress in reducing stress in surgical patients. Ann Surg 2002;236(5):643–8.

[3] Rodgers A, Walker N, Schug S, et al. Reduction of postoperative mortality and morbidity with epidural or spinal anaesthesia: results from overview of randomised trials. Br Med J 2000;321:1–12.

[4] Ross WB, Leaver HA, Yap PL, et al. Immune effects of blood transfusion: macrophage prostaglandin E2 and oxidative responses to endotoxin. Prostaglandins Leucot Essent Fatty Acids 1993;49:945–54.

[5] Payner T, Leaver HA, Knapp B, et al. Microsomal prostaglandin E synthase-1 regulates human glioma cell growth via prostaglandin E2-dependent activation of type II protein kinase A. Mol Cancer Ther 2006;5:1817–26.

[6] Raeburn CD, Sheppard F, Barsness KA, et al. Cytokines for surgeons. Am J Surg 2002;183(3):268–73.

[7] Sato Y, Mukai K, Watanabe S, et al. Lymphocyte subsets in pulmonary venous and arterial blood of lung cancer patients. Jpn J Clin Oncol 1989;19: 229–36.

[8] Zeh HJ, Lotze MT. Addicted to death: invasive cancer and the immune response to unscheduled cell death. J Immunother 2005;28:1–9.

[9] Zou W. Immunosuppressive networks in the tumour environment and their therapeutic relevance. Nat Rev Cancer 2005;5:263–74.

[10] Germenis AE, Karanikas V. Immunoepigenetics: the unseen side of cancer immunoediting. Immunol Cell Biol 2007;85:55–9.

[11] Delves PJ, Martin SJ, Burton DR, et al. Roitt's essential immunology. Oxford (UK): Blackwell Publishing; 2006. p. 384–409.

[12] Leaver HA, Craig SR, Yap PL, et al. Lymphocyte responses following open and minimally invasive thoracic surgery. Eur J Clin Invest 2000;30(3):230–8.

[13] Kehlet H. Surgical stress response: does endoscopic surgery confer an advantage? World J Surg 1999; 23(8):801–7.

[14] Rush S, Khan G, Bamisaiye A, et al. c-jun amino-terminal kinase and mitogen activated protein kinase 1/2 mediate hepatocyte growth factor-induced migration of brain endothelial cells. Exp Cell Res 2007;313:121–32.

[15] Backhus LM. Perioperative cyclooxygenase 2 inhibition to reduce tumor cell adhesion and metastatic potential of circulating tumor cells in non-small cell lung cancer. J Thorac Cardiovasc Surg 2006; 132:297–303.

[16] Tschernko EM, Hofer S, Bieglmayer C, et al. Early postoperative stress: video-assisted wedge resection/lobectomy vs conventional axillary thoracotomy. Chest 1996;109(6):1636–42.

[17] Decker D, Schondorf M, Bidlingmaier F, et al. Surgical stress induces a shift in the type-1/type-2 T-helper cell balance, suggesting down-regulation of cell-mediated and up-regulation of antibody-mediated immunity commensurate to the trauma. Surgery 1996;119(3):316–25.

[18] Brune IB, Wilkie W, Holzmann B, et al. Laparoscopic or open surgery: the role of postoperative immunosuppression in the choice of surgical access. Presented at the 7th International Congress of the European Association for Endoscopic Surgery. Linz, Austria, June 23–26, 1999.

[19] Nishiguchi K, Okuda J, Toyoda M, et al. Comparative evaluation of surgical stress of laparoscopic and open surgeries for colorectal carcinoma. Dis Colon Rectum 2001;44(2):223–30.

[20] Braga M, Vignali A, Gianotti L, et al. Laparoscopic versus open colorectal surgery: a randomized trial on short-term outcome. Ann Surg 2002;236(6): 759–66.

[21] Gebhard FT, Becker HP, Gerngross UB. Reduced inflammatory response in minimal invasive surgery of pneumothorax. Arch Surg 1996;131:1079–82.

[22] Sugi K, Kaneda Y, Esato K. Video-assisted thoracoscopic lobectomy reduces cytokine production more

than conventional open lobectomy. Jpn J Thorac Cardiovasc Surg 2000;48(3):161–5.

[23] Yim AP, Wan S, Lee TW, et al. VATS lobectomy reduces cytokine responses compared with conventional surgery. Ann Thorac Surg 2000;70(1):243–7.

[24] Craig SR, Leaver HA, Yap PL, et al. Acute phase responses following minimal access and conventional thoracic surgery. Eur J Cardiothorac Surg 2001; 20(3):455–63.

[25] Nagahiro I, Andou A, Aoe M, et al. Pulmonary function, postoperative pain, and serum cytokine level after lobectomy: a comparison of VATS and conventional procedure. Ann Thorac Surg 2001; 72(2):362–5.

[26] Kuda T, Kamada Y, Nagamine N, et al. Evaluation of inflammatory-response-induced thoracoscopic surgical stress. Jpn J Thorac Cardiovasc Surg 2002; 50(5):206–9.

[27] Salo M. Effects of anaesthesia and surgery on the immune response. Acta Anaesthesiol Scand 1992;36: 201–20.

[28] McBride WT, Armstrong MA, McBride SJ. Immunomodulation: an important concept in modern anaesthesia. Anaesthesia 1996;51:466–73.

[29] Sugi K, Kaneda Y, Esato K. Video-assisted thoracoscopic lobectomy achieves a satisfactory long-term prognosis in patients with clinical stage IA lung cancer. World J Surg 2000;24(1):27–30; [discussion: 30–1].

[30] Walker WS, Codispoti M, Soon SY, et al. Long-term outcomes following VATS lobectomy for non-small cell bronchogenic carcinoma. Eur J Cardiothorac Surg 2003;23(3):397–402.

[31] Roviaro G, Varoli F, Vergani C, et al. Long-term survival after videothoracoscopic lobectomy for stage I lung cancer. Chest 2004;126(3):725–32.

[32] Shiraishi T, Shirakusa T, Hiratsuka M, et al. Video-assisted thoracoscopic surgery lobectomy for c-T1N0M0 primary lung cancer: its impact on locoregional control. Ann Thorac Surg 2006;82(3): 1021–6.

[33] McKenna RJ Jr, Houck W, Fuller CB. Video-assisted thoracic surgery lobectomy: experience with 1,100 cases. Ann Thorac Surg 2006;81(2):421–5; [discussion: 425–6].

[34] Mocellin S, Rossi CR, Lise M, et al. Adjuvant immunotherapy for solid tumors: from promise to clinical application. Cancer Immunol Immunother 2002;51: 583–95.

[35] Pardoll DM. Spinning molecular immunology into successful immunotherapy. Nat Rev Immunol 2002;2:227–38.

ELSEVIER
SAUNDERS

Thorac Surg Clin 17 (2007) 251–259

THORACIC
SURGERY
CLINICS

Stereotactic Body Radiation Therapy for Stage I Non–Small Cell Lung Cancer

Joe Y. Chang, MD, PhD[a], Jack A. Roth, MD[b],*

[a]Department of Radiation Oncology, The University of Texas MD Anderson Cancer Center,
1515 Holcombe Boulevard, Houston, TX 77030–0097, USA
[b]Department of Thoracic and Cardiovascular Surgery, Unit 445, The University of Texas MD Anderson Cancer Center,
PO Box 301402, Houston, TX 77230–1402, USA

Non–small cell lung cancer (NSCLC) was diagnosed in an estimated 75% of patients with bronchogenic carcinoma in 2006 [1]. Currently, among patients with NSCLC, 15% to 20% present with operable early stage disease [1,2]. The number of diagnoses of early stage (I–II) NSCLC, however, is expected to rise substantially over the next few decades because of the widespread use of screening with spiral CT. Surgical resection is the treatment of choice for these patients and has resulted in 5-year survival rates of 60% to 70% [1,2].

Patients with early stage disease who cannot undergo surgery because of their lung function, cardiac function, bleeding tendency, or other comorbid conditions or who refuse surgery should be considered for definitive radiation therapy. The rate of death from intercurrent disease in this population is quite high. Conventional fractionated radiotherapy (60–66 Gy in 1.8- or 2-Gy fractions) in these patients has resulted in 5-year local control rates of 30% to 50% and overall survival rates of 10% to 30% [3,4]. Modern three-dimensional conformal radiotherapy (3-DCRT), however, may improve clinical outcome compared with two-dimensional radiotherapy [5].

From the basic principles advocated by Fletcher [6], doses ranging from 80 to 100 Gy using 1.8 Gy or 2 Gy per fraction are required to sterilize the tumors frequently treated in patients with bronchogenic carcinoma. Several studies have reported a benefit from such a dose

escalation, suggesting a dose-response relationship from the standpoint of both survival and local disease control in these patients [3,4,7,8]. There are two fundamental problems, however, with the delivery of such doses in patients with lung cancer: the high rate of distant metastases (the major contributor to tumor-related mortality) and the normal tissue toxicity to thoracic organs. Because early stage NSCLC is not inherently a systemic disease at the time of diagnosis and because local control is poor after conventional radiotherapy, research directed toward improving survival should put more emphasis on improving local tumor obliteration.

3-DCRT and hypofractionated stereotactic body radiation therapy (SBRT) allow precise targeting and delivery of radiotherapy. SBRT for lung cancer integrates elements of 3-DCRT with systems for treating tumors in motion and for decreasing setup uncertainty through the use of image-guided radiotherapy techniques. These systems allow the reduction of treatment volumes, facilitate hypofractionation with markedly increased daily doses, and substantially reduce overall treatment time. SBRT combines multiple beam angles to achieve sharp dose gradients, high-precision localization, and a high dose per fraction in extracranial locations. This approach delivers a high biologically effective dose (BED) to the target while minimizing the normal tissue toxicities, which may translate into improved local control and survival rates. The preliminary data have shown greater than 85% local control rates and promising survival rates in patients with stage I NSCLC treated with SBRT. This article

---

* Corresponding author.
  E-mail address: jroth@mdanderso.org (J.A. Roth).

discusses the rationale, indications, optimal BED, and techniques for SBRT compared with surgical resection in patients with stage I NSCLC.

Biologic rationale for hypofractionated stereotactic body radiation therapy

Conventional fractionation (1.8 or 2 Gy per fraction) was based on the "four R" concept of radiobiology: repair of sublethal damage (usually takes 1–6 hours); repopulation (usually 2–4 weeks, depending on specific tissue); reoxygenation (usually 1–3 days, depending on the tumor response); and reassortment of cells within the cell cycle (usually 4–8 hours). The reasoning behind dividing a radiation dose into a number of fractions is that it spares normal tissue; specifically, the resulting sublethal damage can be repaired (more efficiently in normal cells than in cancer cells) and normal tissue can be repopulated between dose fractions. At the same time, fractionated radiotherapy increases the damage to tumor cells because reoxygenation occurs during the tumor response (the hypoxic cell is resistant to radiation) and cells are reassorted into the radiosensitive phases of the cell cycle (cells are most sensitive to radiation at or close to mitosis). Excessively prolonged radiotherapy, however, allows surviving tumor cells to proliferate during treatment. For stage I NSCLC, reoxygenation is less important because of the small size of the cancerous lesion, which is usually well oxygenated. Normal tissue repopulation is also less important if the lesion is not close to critical structures. For these reasons, hypofractionated SBRT with less than 10 fractions is effective and tolerated for stage I NSCLC.

A further consideration in these patients, indeed in any patient treated with radiotherapy, is the cancer killing and radiation-induced effects (eg, esophagitis, pneumonitis, or skin reaction) that occur during or soon after radiation treatment; these are considered acute effects. Radiation-induced effects that occur later (eg, esophageal stricture, fistula, or lung or skin fibrosis) and result in long-term toxicity are considered late effects of radiation. Both the radiation fraction size and the overall treatment time determine the acute effects, whereas the fraction size alone is the dominant determining factor for late effects.

The BED is a well-accepted means of evaluating the acute or late effects of radiation therapy. The BED is calculated with the following linear quadratic equation: $BED = n \times d\,[1 + d/(\alpha/\beta)]$ (where n

is the number of fractions, d is the dose per fraction, and $n \times d$ is the total dose delivered) using an α/β of 10 for acute effects and of 3 for late effects. The higher the BED, the better the chances of eliminating the cancer. There are two ways to increase the BED: delivering a higher total dose by increasing the number of fractions while keeping the conventional dose per fraction, or delivering a higher dose per fraction but lowering the total dose and the number of fractions, which is done in SBRT. The primary concern about SBRT, however, is chronic toxicity.

Radiation-induced toxic effects in normal tissue are related to both the dose and treatment volume. The spatial arrangement of the functional subunits in the normal tissue is also critical. In the case of tissue in which the functional subunits are arranged in a series, such as spinal cord, esophagus, trachea, bronchus, vessels, and nerve, the integrity of each functional subunit is important for organ function, and the elimination of any functional subunits may result in substantial toxicity. In such cases, hot spots, particularly a very high dose to these organs, should be minimized, even for small treatment volumes. In contrast, in tissues such as the lung, in which the functional subunits are arranged in parallel, the integrity of each functional subunit is less important; instead, the volume irradiated or spared plays a major role in the development of complications in these tissues. For stage I NSCLC, image-guided hypofractionated SBRT can deliver a high BED to a cancerous lesion while avoiding critical structures. Such an approach may provide better local control and survival rates with an acceptable toxicity.

Indications for stereotactic body radiation therapy

In general, SBRT should be considered only for early stage (stage I [T1–T2, N0, M0] or selective stage II [T3 with chest wall involvement, N0, M0]) NSCLC. Because the ablative dose is delivered to the target, the target should be away from critical structures, such as the main bronchus, major vessels, trachea, heart, esophagus, spinal cord, and brachial plexus. When an extremely high-dose regimen is used, such as 60 Gy delivered in three fractions, the target should be at least 2 cm away from the bronchial tree (see discussion below). If a milder-dose regimen, such as 50 Gy in four fractions, is used, the 2-cm rule is not required.

Clinical outcome and biologically effective dose considerations

Several studies have shown considerably improved local control and survival rates in patients with stage I lung cancer treated with SBRT. For example, Uematsu and colleagues [9] reported their 5-year experience in patients with stage I NSCLC treated with CT-guided frameless SBRT. Fifty patients were treated with 50 to 60 Gy in 5 to 10 fractions over 1 to 2 weeks. At a median follow-up of 36 months, 6% of patients developed local failure. The 3-year overall survival and disease-specific survival rates were 66% and 88%, respectively. For patients with medically operable disease, however, the 3-year overall survival rate was 88%. No definite adverse effects were noted. Onishi and colleagues [10] reported on the delivery of 60 Gy to the planning target volume (PTV) in 10 fractions (6 Gy per fraction) in patients with stage I NSCLC; 6% of these patients had local progression, and 14% had distant or regional lymph node metastasis. Also, 9% experienced grade 2 or higher toxic effects. The 2-year overall survival rate was 58% in all patients and 83% in those with operable disease. Additionally, Nagata and colleagues [11] reported on the delivery of 48 Gy to the isocenter in four fractions (12 Gy per fraction) over 5 to 13 days in patients with early stage NSCLC. The local control rate was 98% and the 5-year overall survival rate was 83% in patients with stage Ia disease and was 72% in those with stage Ib disease. In about 6.7% of these patients, disease recurred in the regional lymph nodes, and 15% to 20% of patients developed distant metastasis. None of the patients experienced grade 3 or higher toxic effects. In an undergoing multi-institutional phase II study conducted by the Japan Clinical Oncology Group, patients with T1N0M0 NSCLC receive 48 Gy delivered in four fractions to the tumor isocenter. In the United States, Timmerman's group [12] conducted a phase I dose-escalation study using SBRT for patients with stage I NSCLC. These researchers prescribed radiation to the 80% isodose line and escalated the dose from 24 to 72 Gy (delivered in three fractions over 2 weeks). The local failure rate was 21%, and the regional or distant metastasis rate was about 30%. Most of the local failures occurred in patients who received doses of less than or equal to 48 Gy. Grade 3 and higher toxic effects occurred in patients treated with doses of greater than or equal to 48 Gy. Timmerman and

colleagues [13] then conducted a phase II clinical study of 70 patients with stage I inoperable NSCLC treated with SBRT at doses of 60 to 66 Gy in three fractions over 1 to 2 weeks. The median follow-up was 17.5 months; the 2-year local control rate was 95%, and the overall survival rate was 54.7%. Twenty percent of these patients developed grade 3 to 5 toxicity, however, most commonly those with centrally located lesions. This dose regimen is considered too toxic for centrally located tumors and should be used only for peripheral lesions (located at least 2 cm from the bronchial tree). Currently, the Radiation Therapy Oncology Group is conducting a phase 2 clinical study of 60 Gy delivered in three fractions (as described by Timmerman and colleagues [13]) in patients with inoperable stage I and selective stage II peripherally located NSCLC. Recently, Xia and colleagues [14] reported results from a phase II study of SBRT in 43 patients with medically inoperable stage I to II peripherally or centrally located NSCLC. When 70 Gy was delivered at 7 Gy per fraction to the gross tumor volume (GTV), the 1-, 2-, and 3-year local control rates were 95% in all patients. The 1-, 2-, and 3-year overall survival rates were 100%, 91%, and 91%, respectively, in patients with stage I disease and 73%, 64%, and 64%, respectively, in those with stage II disease. Only 2.3% (1 of 43) of the patients had grade 3 pneumonitis [14].

The optimal dose and fractionation for SBRT is unclear. Onishi and colleagues [15] retrospectively evaluated results from a Japanese multi-institutional SBRT study. At a total of 13 institutions, 245 patients with stage I NSCLC were treated with hypofractionated high-dose SBRT. A total dose of 18 to 75 Gy at the isocenter was administered in 1 to 22 fractions. The median calculated BED was 108 Gy (range, 57–180 Gy), and the median follow-up was 24 months. Greater than grade 2 pulmonary complications were observed in only six patients (2.4%). The local recurrence rate was 8.1% for those given a BED of greater than or equal to 100 Gy, but was 26.4% when the BED was less than 100 Gy ($P < .05$). The 5-year overall survival rate in patients with medically operable NSCLC was 88.4% for those given a BED of greater than or equal to 100 Gy, compared with 69.4% when the BED was less than 100 Gy ($P < .05$). NSCLC recurred in the regional lymph nodes in 8.2% of patients, and distant metastasis occurred in 14.7% of patients. Recently, Onishi and colleagues updated their results at a median follow-up of 38 months. At 5 years, the local failure rate was 8.4% and the overall survival rate was 72% for patients with operable disease who received SBRT with a BED of greater than 100 Gy (2006 SBRT workshop in Maui, Hawaii, sponsored by the International Association for the Study of Lung Cancer, unpublished data). Their data showed that hypofractionated high-dose SBRT with a BED less than 180 Gy was feasible and beneficial for the curative treatment of patients with stage I NSCLC. For all treatment methods and schedules, local control and survival rates were better in patients treated with a BED of greater than or equal to 100 Gy than with a BED of less than 100 Gy. Survival rates in patients with medically operable disease treated with a BED of greater than or equal to 100 Gy were comparable with those of patients who underwent surgery.

The BED, calculated with the linear quadratic equation using an α/β of 10, was 96 Gy with the delivery of 60 Gy in 10 fractions, 106 Gy with the delivery of 48 Gy in four fractions, 119 Gy with the delivery of 70 Gy in 10 fractions, and 180 Gy with the delivery of 60 Gy in three fractions. When one considers the optimal BED for SBRT, however, one also needs to keep in mind the potential long-term toxicity associated with SBRT, particularly for lesions close to critical structures, such as the trachea, bronchus, vessels, nerves, esophagus, spinal cord, heart, and skin. The current consensus is that the BED must be greater than 100 Gy and that the volume of the critical structures receiving the high BED (>80 Gy) should be minimized. In general, only peripherally located disease should be treated with SBRT. When SBRT is used for patients with a centrally located tumor without further long-term toxicity data, a greater number of fractions or a lower BED should be considered.

Stereotactic body radiation therapy techniques

SBRT required sophisticated 3-DCRT, image-guided radiation therapy and reliable immobilization device. Several techniques have been reported previously. Techniques using the linear accelerator–based 3-DCRT with daily imaging are now discussed.

Immobilization and tumor motion consideration

Immobilization is crucial in SBRT to reduce daily setup uncertainty. The appropriate immobilization should be chosen for each patient. The authors immobilize patients in an arms-up position using a commercially available vacuum immobilization bag, which extends from the patient's head to the pelvis, combined with a wing board.

Consideration of tumor motion in SBRT is very critical in patients whose tumor moves substantially during radiotherapy. In a recent four-dimensional CT (4-DCT) study of 72 patients with lung cancer, Liu and colleagues [16] showed tumor movement of more than 1 cm during breathing in 13% of the patients, particularly in those with small lower lobe tumors close to the diaphragm. An individualized tumor-motion margin should be considered for such patients. In addition, patients should be evaluated for regularity of breathing, responsiveness to feedback guidance, and breath-holding capability. On the basis of this evaluation, one of the following treatment-delivery techniques can be selected: (1) free-breathing approach (with or without feedback guidance); (2) respiratory-gated approach; (3) breath-holding approach (with or without feedback guidance); (4) abdominal compression; or (5) a combination of these techniques.

For patients with tumor motion of less than 5 mm, simple expansion of the tumor-motion margin is adequate (free-breathing approach). For patients with considerable tumor motion, however, particularly movement of greater than 1 cm, an individualized tumor-motion margin should be considered. A commercially available system can be used for these patients by respiratory-gated approach [17]. This technique uses an externally placed fiducial that is tracked as the patient breathes. The beam can be triggered at a chosen point in the respiratory cycle; this is typically done at the end of expiration because this is the longest and most reproducible portion of the respiratory cycle. This technique requires patients to be able to breathe slowly in a regular pattern. Active breathing control and deep-inspiration breath-holding are two techniques that have been pioneered to help patients hold their breaths at reproducible points in the respiratory cycle [18,19]. The radiation beam is then initiated. These two techniques limit patient respiratory excursion to fixed volumes, and they limit diaphragm excursion to about 5 mm instead of 10 to 15 mm. These techniques, however, require very cooperative patients who are able to hold their breath for at least 15 seconds. Abdominal compression has been used in some institutions to reduce the diaphragm movement.

With the advent of new technologies, such as multislice detectors and faster imaging reconstruction, it is now possible to image real-time breathing and to assess organ motion using 4-DCT [20]. 4-DCT is a fast CT technique that can capture the tumor positions during the whole breathing cycle. With 4-DCT, the patient can be scanned in each couch position for the whole breathing cycle (usually 5–6 seconds in each position) and then moved to the next couch position. After scanning, the computer re-sorts all of the images and reconstructs the tumor positions for the whole breathing cycle, thereby providing a movie-like picture of the tumor motion. Because of these capabilities, 4-DCT simulation is recommended for SBRT. If 4-DCT is not available, other methods of determining tumor motion should be applied [9,12].

Stereotactic body radiation therapy target volume delineation

The International Commission on Radiological Units and Measurements Report No. 50 provides guidelines [21] for defining targets in the treatment of lung cancer. The GTV is the primary tumor and any grossly involved lymph nodes. The clinical tumor volume is the anatomically defined area believed to harbor micrometastasis (hilar or mediastinal lymph nodes or a margin around the grossly visible disease). The PTV accounts for physiologic organ motion during treatment and the inaccuracies of daily setup in fractionated therapy. In the International Commission on Radiological Units and Measurements Report No. 62, a new concept of the internal target volume was proposed as the volume encompassing the clinical tumor volume and the internal margin to compensate for expected physiologic movements and the variations in size, shape, and position of the clinical tumor volume during radiotherapy.

Gross tumor volume

The GTV should be delineated using CT. The pulmonary extent of lung tumors should be delineated on lung windows. Positron emission tomography (PET) should be used only for disease staging.

Internal gross target volume

If 4-DCT is available, the internal gross target volume (IGTV), which is the volume containing the GTV throughout its motion during respiration, can be designed. One method of combining the data from the multiple CT datasets is to create a maximal intensity projection, which can be used as an aid in contouring the IGTV. Another approach is to use deformable registration technique in which the tumor volume that is outlined on the expiratory phase of the four-dimensional images is registered on other phases of the images to create a union of target contours, enclosing all possible positions of the target. The third approach is to contour the GTV with inspiration and expiration breath-holding and then combine these two volumes to form IGTV. The last approach can be used with regular spiral CT without four dimensions. All CT datasets are transferred to the treatment-planning system for reference.

Clinical target volume

The clinical tumor volume consists of the GTV plus an 8-mm margin that is edited as necessary to account for physical boundaries.

Internal target volume

The internal target volume consists of an IGTV plus an 8-mm margin that is edited as appropriate.

Planning target volume

The PTV consists of either a clinical tumor volume plus a margin for tumor motion and for daily setup uncertainty or an internal target volume plus a margin for daily setup uncertainty.

Onboard imaging

Daily onboard imaging, such as CT on-rail simulation, cone beam CT, or four-dimensional cone beam CT, are recommended during each fraction of radiotherapy. For each day of the imaging study, the position of the target should be adjusted and the target coverage should be confirmed. The setup uncertainty can be kept to less than 3 mm using the daily CT on-rail image. If daily CT is not available, a larger setup margin is advised.

Image-guided stereotactic body radiation therapy at MD Anderson Cancer Center

Currently at The University of Texas MD Anderson Cancer Center, all patients with early stage NSCLC undergo 4-DCT simulation for SBRT, and daily on-board imaging, such as CT on-rail simulation, to determine tumor motion and daily setup variation. Preliminary data of image-guided SBRT in patients with early stage

NSCLC were reported [22]. Thirty-seven patients with pathologically confirmed stage I disease were treated with SBRT. NSCLC in all patients was staged with chest CT, PET, and brain MRI. 4-DCT images were obtained with a GE simulator with the Varian RPM system (Varian Medical System, Inc., Palo Alto, California). The IGTV was delineated using a maximal intensity projection that was created by combining the data from the multiple 4-DCT datasets at different breath phases. The internal target volume consisted of the IGTV plus an 8-mm margin, and a 3-mm setup uncertainty margin was added to form the PTV. Daily CT on-rail simulation was conducted during each fraction of radiotherapy. SBRT was prescribed at a dose of 50 Gy to the PTV, delivered at 12.5 Gy per fraction for 4 consecutive days (the BED was 112.5 Gy). Critical structures, such as the main bronchus, heart, and major vessels, were excluded from the 40-Gy isodose line. Patients were followed-up with chest CT every 3 months for 2 years. PET follow-up was recommended at 3 to 5 months after SBRT.

The progression-free survival rate at the treatment site in all patients was 100%, with a median follow-up of 10 months [22]. The complete response rate was 100% in 11 patients who underwent PET for post-SBRT evaluation. The rate of stable disease was 4.5%. Mediastinal lymph node metastasis and distant metastasis developed in 4% of patients. There was no grade 2 or higher radiation-induced pneumonitis in patients with stage I disease, and no esophagitis was noted. Grade II to III dermatitis developed at the treatment site in 9.5% of patients. All patients tolerated SBRT well, with no symptoms of toxicity during SBRT. More studies with long-term patient follow-up are needed. Fig. 1 shows a representative patient with stage I NSCLC who received SBRT and achieved a complete clinical response.

Omitting prophylactic lymph node irradiation

For many years, standard radiation therapy in the United States, with some recent exceptions, consisted of 40 to 50 Gy delivered to electively irradiated regional-nodal areas (ipsilateral, contralateral, hilar, mediastinal, and occasionally supraclavicular), with an additional 20 Gy delivered to the primary tumor through reduced fields. This regimen was based on pathologic information regarding the high incidence of hilar and mediastinal node metastases in patients with

bronchogenic carcinoma. The rationale opposing elective nodal irradiation has been the high local recurrence rates within the previously irradiated tumor volume and the high likelihood of distant metastasis; the thinking was that if gross disease cannot be controlled, why enlarge the irradiated volumes to include areas that may harbor microscopic disease?

Three major factors have changed the standards for radiation therapy in recent years: (1) the use of chemotherapy, (2) the advent of 3-DCRT, and (3) better disease staging and target delineation with PET. In addition, emerging clinical data have shown that omitting prophylactic lymph node irradiation does not reduce the local control rate for patients receiving definitive radiotherapy, who have isolated outside-field (field of radiotherapy) local recurrence rates of 3% to 8%, particularly in patients with stage I disease and in those who undergo PET for disease staging [23–25].

About 15% to 20% of patients with stage I NSCLC who receive SBRT developed distant metastasis, more commonly in those with T2 disease. In recent studies of adjuvant chemotherapy after surgical resection for early stage NSCLC, there was a 4% to 15% survival benefit in patients with stage Ib NSCLC or higher who received postoperative chemotherapy [26–28]. Adjuvant chemotherapy after SBRT should be considered in T2 disease if the patient can tolerate it.

Comparison of stereotactic body radiation therapy with surgical resection in operable stage I non–small cell lung cancer

The role of SBRT in operable stage I NSCLC remains unclear. Currently, lobectomy with mediastinal sampling or dissection is considered the standard treatment for this disease. Supporting this were the findings from a study conducted by the Lung Cancer Study Group [29], which consisted of a randomized comparison of an anatomic lobectomy versus limited (wedge or segmental) resection for peripheral T1 pulmonary carcinomas. The locoregional recurrence rate associated with limited resection was three times greater than that associated with lobectomy, 17% versus 6.4%. The potential advantages of surgical resection include the complete removal of the involved lobe, resulting in less chance of local recurrence, and the pathologic stage (maybe therapeutic in some cases) of hilar or mediastinal lymph nodes. If a lymph node is involved,

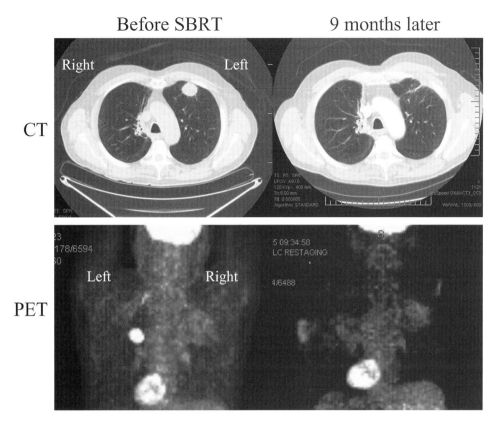

Fig. 1. A representative patient with stage I NSCLC who received SBRT (50 Gy in four fractions) and achieved a complete clinical response.

adjuvant chemotherapy or radiotherapy (for N2 disease) may be considered.

The 5-year overall survival rate for patients with medically operable stage I NSCLC treated with SBRT is about 70%, which is comparable with surgical data from Japan [30] and the United States. Follow-up in all of these series, however, is still relatively short. SBRT avoids the operative mortality and postoperative complications associated with surgery. High-volume centers, however, now achieve operative mortality rates of less than 1% [31]. Multi-institutional phase II studies of SBRT for potentially resectable stage I NSCLC have begun in Japan (JCOG0403) and the United States (RTOG0236).

Clinical data indicated an improved therapeutic ratio for SBRT in patients with inoperable stage I NSCLC. Comparable data for patients with operable disease, however, are scarce. To determine the role of SBRT in patients with operable stage I NSCLC, a randomized study is warranted. This was the topic of a recent workshop held by the International Association for the Study of Lung Cancer. This trial requires about 1000 patients and needs to be international in scope to be successful. It was clear from the conference presentations that SBRT technology had reached a point where this comparison is both feasible and justified if the appropriate roles of SBRT and surgery in the treatment of early stage lung cancer are to be determined.

Summary

Image-guided SBRT with the delivery of a BED greater than 100 Gy is feasible and safe in the treatment of peripherally located inoperable stage I NSCLC. The 3- to 5-year local control and overall survival rates for SBRT seem to be much better than the rates for conventional radiotherapy, and the toxicity rate is minimal. Particularly for stage Ia (T1N0M0) disease, survival rates with SBRT were comparable with rates seen with surgical resection. SBRT is becoming the standard treatment for inoperable stage I NSCLC. Its role in operable stage I NSCLC, however, is not clear.

To balance improved targeting accuracy with minimized treatment-related toxicity, a reliable immobilization device and consideration of image-guided tumor motion are crucial. The optimal dose regimen remains unclear, but a BED greater than 100 Gy seems warranted.

References

[1] Jemal A, Siegel R, Ward E, et al. Cancer statistics. CA Cancer J Clin 2006;56(2):106–30.

[2] Mountain C. The international system for staging lung cancer. Semin Surg Oncol 2000;18(2):106–15.

[3] Dosoretz D, Galmarini D, Rubenstein J, et al. Local control in medically inoperable lung cancer: an analysis of its importance in outcome and factors determining the probability of tumor eradication. Int J Radiat Oncol Biol Phys 1993;27:507–16.

[4] Kaskowitz L, Graham M, Emami B, et al. Radiation therapy alone for stage I non-small cell lung cancer. Int J Radiat Oncol Biol Phys 1993;27:517–23.

[5] Fang L, Komaki R, Allen P, et al. Comparison of outcomes for patients with medically inoperable stage I non-small-cell lung cancer treated with two-dimensional vs. three-dimensional radiotherapy. Int J Radiat Oncol Biol Phys 2006;66(1): 108–16.

[6] Fletcher G. Clinical dose response curves of human malignant epithelial tumours. Br J Cancer 1973;46: 1–12.

[7] Dosoretz D, Katin M, Blitzer P, et al. Medically inoperable lung carcinoma: the role of radiation therapy. Semin Radiat Oncol 1996;6:98–104.

[8] Sibley G, Jamieson T, Marks L, et al. Radiotherapy alone for medically inoperable stage I non-small-cell lung cancer: the Duke experience. Int J Radiat Oncol Biol Phys 1998;40(1):149–54.

[9] Uematsu M, Shioda A, Suda A, et al. Computed tomography-guided frameless stereotactic radiotherapy for stage I non-small cell lung cancer: a 5-year experience. Int J Radiat Oncol Biol Phys 2001; 51(3):666–70.

[10] Onishi H, Kuriyama K, Komiyama T, et al. Clinical outcomes of stereotactic radiotherapy for stage I non-small cell lung cancer using a novel irradiation technique: patient self-controlled breath-hold and beam switching using a combination of linear accelerator and CT scanner. Lung Cancer 2004;45(1): 45–55.

[11] Nagata Y, Takayama K, Matsuo Y, et al. Clinical outcomes of a phase I/II study of 48 Gy of stereotactic body radiotherapy in 4 fractions for primary lung cancer using a stereotactic body frame. Int J Radiat Oncol Biol Phys 2005;63(5):1427–31.

[12] McGarry R, Papiez L, Williams M, et al. Stereotactic body radiation therapy of early-stage non-small-cell lung carcinoma: Phase I study. Int J Radiat Oncol Biol Phys 2005;63(4):1010–5.

[13] Timmerman R, McGarry R, Yiannoutsos C, et al. Excessive toxicity when treating central tumors in a phase II study of stereotactic body radiation therapy for medically inoperable early-stage lung cancer. J Clin Oncol 2006;24(30):4833–9.

[14] Xia T, Li H, Sun Q, et al. Promising clinical outcome of stereotactic body radiation therapy for patients with inoperable stage I/II non-small-cell lung cancer. Int J Radiat Oncol Biol Phys 2006;66: 117–25.

[15] Onishi H, Araki T, Shirato H, et al. Stereotactic hypofractionated high-dose irradiation for stage I non-small cell lung carcinoma clinical outcome in 245 subjects in a Japanese multiinstitutional study. Cancer 2004;101(7):1623–31.

[16] Liu H, Choi B, Zhang J, et al. Assessing respiration-induced tumor motion and margin of internal target volume for image-guided radiotherapy of lung cancers. Int J Radiat Oncol Biol Phys 2005;63(Suppl 1):S30–S3S.

[17] Ramsey C, Scaperoth D, Arwood D, et al. Clinical efficacy of respiratory gated conformal radiation therapy. Med Dosim 1999;24(2):115–9.

[18] Rosenzweig K, Hanley J, Mah D, et al. The deep inspiration breath-hold technique in the treatment of inoperable non-small-cell lung cancer. Int J Radiat Oncol Biol Phys 2000;48(1):81–7.

[19] Sixel K, Aznar M, Ung Y. Deep inspiration breath hold to reduce irradiated heart volume in breast cancer patients. Int J Radiat Oncol Biol Phys 2001; 49(1):199–204.

[20] Nehmeh S, Erdi Y, Pan T, et al. Four-dimensional (4D) PET/CT imaging of the thorax. Med Phys 2004;31:3179–86.

[21] International Commission on Radiation Units and Measurements. Prescribing, recording, and reporting photon beam therapy. Bethesda (MD); 1993. Report No.: 50.

[22] Chang J, Balter P, Liao Z, et al. Preliminary report of image-guided hypofractionated stereotactic body radiotherapy to treat patients with medically inoperable stage I or isolated peripheral lung recurrent non-small cell lung cancer. Int J Radiat Oncol Biol Phys 2006;66(3):S480.

[23] Bradley J, Thorstad W, Mutic S, et al. Impact of FDG-PET on radiation therapy volume delineation in non-small-cell lung cancer. Int J Radiat Oncol Biol Phys 2004;59(1):78–86.

[24] Krol A, Aussems P, Noordijk E, et al. Local irradiation alone for peripheral stage I lung cancer: could we omit the elective regional nodal irradiation? Int J Radiat Oncol Biol Phys 1996;34(2):297–302.

[25] Sulman E, Chang J, Liao Z, et al. Exclusion of elective nodal irradiation does not decrease local regional control of non-small cell lung cancer. Int J Radiat Oncol Biol Phys 2005;63(Suppl 1): S226–7.

[26] Winton T, Livingston R, Johnson D, et al. Vinorelbine plus cisplatin vs. observation in resected

non-small-cell lung cancer. N Engl J Med 2005; 352(25):2589–97.

[27] Strauss G, Herndon J, Maddaus M, et al. Randomized clinical trial of adjuvant chemotherapy with paclitaxel and carboplatin following resection in stage IB non-small cell lung cancer (NSCLC): report of cancer and leukemia group B (CALGB) protocol 9633. J Clin Oncol 2004; 22(14):7019.

[28] Arriagada R, Bergman B, Dunant A, et al. Cisplatin-based adjuvant chemotherapy in patients with completely resected non-small-cell lung cancer. N Engl J Med 2004;350(4):351–60.

[29] Ginsberg R, Rubinstein L, Lung Cancer Study Group. Randomized trial of lobectomy versus limited resection for T1 N0 non-small cell lung cancer. Ann Thorac Surg 1995;60:615–22.

[30] Naruke T, Tsuchiya R, Kondo H, et al. Prognosis and survival after resection for bronchogenic carcinoma based on the 1997 TNM-staging classification: the Japanese experience. Ann Thorac Surg 2001; 71(6):1759–64.

[31] Allen MS, Darling GE, Pechet TT, et al. Resections in patients with early-stage lung cancer: initial results of the randomized, prospective ACOSOG Z0030 trial. Ann Thorac Surg 2006;81:1013–20.

THORACIC
SURGERY
CLINICS

Thorac Surg Clin 17 (2007) 261–271

Ablative Treatments for Lung Tumors: Radiofrequency Ablation, Stereotactic Radiosurgery, and Microwave Ablation

Ghulam Abbas, MD, Matthew J. Schuchert, MD, Arjun Pennathur, MD, Sebastien Gilbert, MD, James D. Luketich, MD*

Heart, Lung, and Esophageal Surgery Institute, University of Pittsburgh Medical Center, 200 Lothrop Street, Pittsburgh, PA 15213, USA

The incidence of lung cancer continues to increase with approximately 175,000 new cases diagnosed annually in the United States. Lung cancer remains the number one cause of cancer-related deaths in men and women [1]. Although surgical resection remains the mainstay of therapy for early stage non–small cell lung cancer (NSCLC), most patients present with advanced disease. In addition, many patients with resectable early stage disease are unable to tolerate pulmonary resection because of compromised cardiopulmonary function [2].

External beam radiation therapy remains an option for those patients who are deemed to be at high-risk for pulmonary resection. Treatment results in this setting, however, are inferior to resection and the chance for cure is small. In a study of 71 node-negative patients who received at least 60 Gy of external beam radiation to their primary tumors, 3- and 5-year survivals were only 19% and 12%, respectively [3]. In a recent report of radiation therapy in 60 patients with stage I or II NSCLC, local progression occurred in 53% of patients with a median progression-free survival of 18.5 months and an overall median survival of 20 months [4]. In addition to the disappointing results with external beam radiation, morbidity related to this treatment modality is common. Radiation pneumonitis is a potentially life-threatening problem, particularly for a patient with severely impaired pulmonary function who is not a resection candidate (ie, the usual patient referred for nonoperative therapy). In the series described previously, radiation pneumonitis occurred in 8.3% of patients treated with definitive radiotherapy [4].

New alternatives to standard external beam radiation therapy are now entering clinical practice for the treatment of lung cancer or limited pulmonary metastases in medically inoperable patients. The two principal modalities that are being offered by many centers around the world are radiofrequency ablation (RFA) and stereotactic radiosurgery (SRS). Another ablative modality, microwave ablation (MWA), is also being introduced into practice, although current clinical experience is very limited with this new approach. This article reviews these therapies and discusses their role in the treatment of thoracic malignancies.

Radiofrequency ablation

Technology and mechanism of action

RFA involves the application of high-frequency alternating current to heat and coagulate target lesions. RFA systems have three components: (1) a generator; (2) an active electrode that is placed within the tumor; and (3) a dispersive electrode (bovie pad) placed on the thighs of the patient (Fig. 1). As the radiofrequency energy moves from the active electrode to the dispersive electrode and then back to the active electrode,

* Corresponding author.
  E-mail address: luketichjd@upmc.edu
(J.D. Luketich).

1547-4127/07/$ - see front matter © 2007 Elsevier Inc. All rights reserved.
doi:10.1016/j.thorsurg.2007.03.007

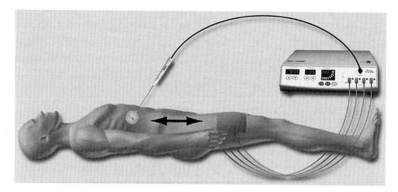

Fig. 1. Components of RFA system; active electrode in tumor, dispersive electrodes (bovie pads), and generator.

ions within the tissue oscillate, resulting in frictional heating of the tissue. As the temperature within the tissue rises to greater than 60°C, instantaneous cell death occurs because of protein denaturation and coagulation necrosis.

The greatest experience with RFA has been achieved in the treatment of liver tumors, both as an adjunct to resection and as primary therapy. Because of a lower rate of complications, RFA has largely replaced other less invasive modalities (eg, cryotherapy) [5,6]. A large international, multicenter study of 2320 patients who received percutaneous RFA for liver malignancies reported a mortality of only 0.3%, and an overall complication rate of 7.1% [7]. Several centers around the world have now published reports of RFA for the lung. These reports primarily demonstrate the safety and feasibility of this technique for lung tumors [8,9].

Animal models have been used to investigate the feasibility of this technique in treating lung tumors, and have helped in the development of the treatment algorithms for humans. In a study by Goldberg and colleagues [10] using a rabbit model of lung sarcoma, seven lesions were treated with RFA for 6 minutes at 90°C, and the remaining four tumors were untreated as controls. The authors noted CT evidence of coagulation necrosis surrounding the tumor, manifested radiologically by increased opacity enveloping the lesion. This was followed temporally by the development of central tissue attenuation consistent with cavitation. Histologic analysis revealed that at least 95% of the tumor nodules were necrotic, although some rabbits (43%) had residual tumor nests at the periphery of the tumor. Pneumothorax was the only procedure-related complication, and occurred in 29% of treated rabbits and in 25% of

controls. In another study, Miao and colleagues [11] implanted VX2 sarcomas in the lung of 18 rabbits (12 treated and 6 controls), and the lesions were then treated with RFA using a cooled-tip electrode for 60 seconds. Absolute tumor eradication was achieved with RFA in 33% of the rabbits. A partial response was observed in 41.6% of rabbits that survived longer than 3 months. On histopathologic evaluation, the ablated lesions retained their fundamental tissue architecture with evidence of coagulation necrosis. Surrounding edema and inflammation was noted in the normal adjacent lung. After 1 to 3 months of treatment, the ablated tumor became an atrophied nodule of coagulation necrosis within a fibrotic capsule. The timing and progression of these postablation changes becomes an important issue when evaluating postprocedure treatment responses.

Some investigators have performed RFA followed by resection to evaluate the efficacy of the ablation procedure within the resected specimen. In one multicenter study of 15 patients, ablation was possible in 13 cases [12]. In these 13 patients median tumor kill was 70%, with seven patients achieving 100% ablation. There seemed to be a learning curve effect with five of the last six cases achieving 100% ablation. More recently, Nguyen and colleagues [13] published the results of an "ablate and resect" study where vital stains were used to assess tumor cell viability. In seven tumors studied with this technique greater than 80% nonviability was demonstrated. Only three patients (38%) demonstrated 100% nonviability in their ablated tumors. All three tumors were less than 2 cm in diameter. It should be noted, however, that a single ablation with either a 3- or 3.5-cm active electrode was performed, so that some of the larger tumors may have been inadequately ablated. These studies demonstrate that although RFA can produce effective ablation, 100% cell death is not achieved in every case.

Currently, there are three Food and Drug Administration–approved devices available within the United States for the performance of RFA: (1) Boston Scientific (Boston, MA), (2) RITA (Mountainview, CA), and (3) Valley Laboratory (Boulder City, CO). The Boston Scientific device is an impedance-based system where the end point of treatment is determined by a significant rise in tissue impedance, indicating that the tumor has been ablated and unable to maintain further conduction. The RITA and Valley Laboratory systems are temperature-based devices, which elevate the tumor temperature to high levels for a designated period of time. The Boston Scientific and RITA active probes both consist of an expandable needle system (Fig. 2), whereas the Valley Laboratory system consists of either a single needle or three parallel needles that are placed within the tumor. The Valley Laboratory electrode consists of a proximal insulated portion and a distal uninsulated active tip. The electrode is irrigated with a continuous infusion of ice-water, and for this reason is sometimes referred to as a "cool-tip" electrode. There has been one animal study that has demonstrated success of these probes both in vivo and ex vivo in pig and calf livers [14]. Currently, no clinical studies have evaluated differences between these probes.

Patient selection

For NSCLC, RFA can be used for stage I patients who are believed to be at increased risk for pulmonary resection, or for those who refuse surgery. Surgical resection may be beneficial for a patient who has more advanced cancer (eg, satellite nodules) localized to the lung [15].

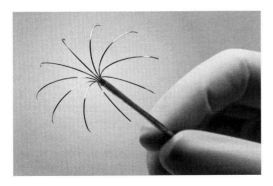

Fig. 2. Boston Scientific electrode.

Occasionally, RFA may be a reasonable therapy for a medically inoperable patient with more advanced cancer (eg, satellite nodules) localized to the lung. The efficacy of RFA is low for nodules greater than 5 cm in diameter [16]. RFA is also not recommended for lesions abutting the mediastinum. Other patients who may be considered for treatment with RFA include those with advanced-stage disease who have responded to definitive radiation and chemotherapy but have a persistent solitary peripheral focus of cancer, and those who present with a recurrent isolated cancer after previous lung resection.

RFA is also a suitable option for some patients with limited peripheral pulmonary metastases. As with resection, this treatment should be reserved for those patients with a limited number of metastases, disease localized to the chest, and with their primary cancer either controlled or controllable. Similar to primary lung cancer, RFA should be reserved for those patients who are believed to be at increased operative risk for resection of their pulmonary metastases. In some situations, complete resection of all pulmonary metastases is not possible, and RFA can be used as an adjunct intraoperatively. The authors have certainly found RFA to be of use in the situation where a wedge resection of a peripheral nodule was performed and resection of other nodules would have required a lobectomy or pneumonectomy. To preserve pulmonary parenchyma, some of these tumors were treated with RFA. Box 1 outlines suggested selection criteria for the use of RFA.

Operative technique

Initially, RFA was performed using an open thoracotomy. Although this approach provides the most controlled method for RFA application, few patients are candidates for treatment this way, because resection is preferable in most situations when thoracotomy is used. Situations may arise, however, such as that described previously where a patient presents with two or more tumors, some amenable to treatment with RFA and other tumors that can be treated with resection. Although video-assisted thoracoscopic surgery has been postulated to be an attractive approach for RFA, optimal needle deployment within the tumor in the setting of a collapsed lung is often difficult to obtain.

The most common method of pulmonary RFA uses a percutaneous CT-guided approach. Either

Box 1. Selection criteria for the use of radiofrequency ablation

Inclusion criteria
Stage I or II[a] NSCLC; poor surgical
    candidate
NSCLC stage IIIb (satellite nodule same
    lobe) or stage IV (nodule in another
    lobe or lung); poor surgical candidate
Stage IIIa or IV with solitary pulmonary
    nodule remaining after standard
    therapies
Pulmonary metastases; primary disease
    controlled or controllable; poor
    surgical candidate
Target lesion 5 cm or less

Exclusion criteria
Tumor abutting hilum or large
    pulmonary vessel
Malignant effusion
Pulmonary hypertension
Greater than three tumors in one lung
Target lesion greater than 5 cm

―――――
    [a] Patients with stage II should receive addi-
tional therapy because N1 disease is not
treated with RFA.

general or local anesthesia can be used when
performing CT-guided RFA. The authors' preference has been to use general anesthesia. This
allows needle deployment, ablation, and biopsies
(if required) to be performed in a more controlled

manner. Additionally, some patients with cardiopulmonary compromise may have difficulty in
lying flat for a prolonged period while awake or
under conscious sedation. Patient positioning is
very important during CT-guided RFA. The
authors prefer to position the patient in such
a way that the target lesion is accessed with
minimal penetration of normal lung parenchyma.
This decreases the risk of hemorrhage and prolonged air leak. Positioning is also important to
ensure adequate clearance of the RFA probe
within the scanner. The maximum number of
lesions that can be ablated in a single setting is
debatable. As a general rule, however, ablation of
more than two to three lesions in one setting is not
recommended.

Treatment response

Following RFA there is an inflammatory response, which may persist for up to 3 months,
making it difficult to determine whether the mass
represents scar or viable cancer. For this reason
the mass may initially appear larger on radiographic imaging, and then subsequently start to
decrease in size with time. Ablated lesions may
demonstrate central cavitation (Fig. 3) or develop
bubble lucencies, which are indicative of effective
ablation.

Other centers have been using CT densitometry protocols to help evaluate for persistent or
recurrent disease [17]. Densitometry involves the
injection of contrast and then obtaining CT images of the ablated nodule at 0, 45, 180, and 300
seconds following the contrast injection. Lesions

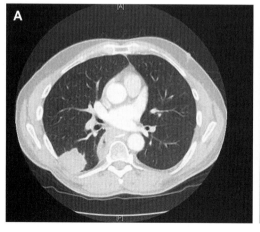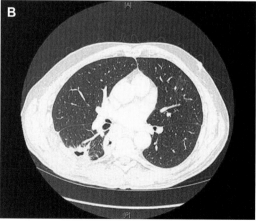

Fig. 3. (*A*) Right lower lobe tumor before RFA. (*B*) Right lower lobe tumor 4 months after RFA.

greater than 9 mm in size that enhance at 15 HU or greater after 1 minute are suspicious for cancer. These densitometry techniques are time consuming, and are typically only valuable for those patients with single tumor nodules. The authors have modified the Response Evaluation Criteria in Solid Tumors to evaluate treatment responses objectively (Table 1) [18]. CT scans are obtained at 3-month intervals looking for evidence of tumor growth. Whenever possible, positron emission tomography scans are also obtained to help in the determination of tumor response.

The American College of Surgeons Oncology Group is opening a multicenter study evaluating RFA in high-risk patients with stage Ia NSCLC in 2006. This study (Z4033) will address such issues as response assessment by standardizing the follow-up protocol in the various study sites. Follow-up assessment will include CT (size criteria and densitometry) and serial positron emission tomography scans.

Clinical results

In their initial experience with RFA, the authors treated 33 tumors in 18 patients [15]. Tumor pathologies included metastatic carcinoma (N = 8); sarcoma (N = 5); and NSCLC (N = 5). The mean age was 60 (range, 27–95) years. The principal finding from this study was the lack of effectiveness in treating tumors greater than 5 cm in size. Using the Response Evaluation Criteria in Solid Tumors they found a radiographically determined response rate of 66% for tumors less or equal to 5 cm in size, compared

with only 33% in patients with tumors greater than 5 cm.

A multicenter study summarizing the results of 493 patients undergoing RFA of pulmonary nodules concluded that RFA was safe, with negligible morbidity and mortality (0.4%), and is associated with a gain in quality of life [19].

The authors have also reported the results of RFA in 18 patients with NSCLC [18]. A total of 21 tumors were treated. Most patients (N = 9) had stage I NSCLC. There were four patients with stage IV cancer. This included three patients with recurrences after previous lobectomy and one patient with a synchronous liver metastasis that was also treated with RFA. The median tumor diameter was 2.8 (range, 1.2–4.5) cm. Although morbidity occurred in 55.6% of patients, this was minor in most cases. The most common complication was a pneumothorax (38.9%), which resolved with pigtail catheter drainage within 24 hours in most cases. At a median follow-up of 14 months, 83.3% of the patients were alive. Local progression occurred in 38.1% of the ablated nodules. For stage I cancer, the mean progression-free interval was 17.6 months; the median progression-free interval was not reached. Although this is a small study, these results compare favorably with standard methods of external beam radiation where local progression is seen in over 50% of cases [4].

More recently, the authors presented their experience with RFA for the treatment of stage I NSCLCs [20]. Nineteen patients underwent RFA over a 3-year period. Median age was 78 years (range, 68–88). An initial complete response was

Table 1
Modified response evaluation criteria in solid tumors for objective evaluation of treatment responses

Response	CT mass size	CT mass quality	PET
Complete (two of the following)	Lesion disappearance (scar) less than 25% of original size	Cyst or cavity formation, low density entire lesion	SUV[a] <2.5
Partial (one of the following)	More than 30% decrease in the LD of target lesion	Central necrosis or central cavitation with liquid density	Decreased SUV or area of FDG uptake
Stable lesion (one of the following)	Less than 30% decrease in the LD of target lesion	Mass solid appearance, no central necrosis or cavitation	Unchanged SUV or area of FDG uptake
Progression (two of the following)	Increase of more than 20% in the LD of target lesion	Solid mass, invasion adjacent structures	Higher SUV or larger area of FDG uptake

Abbreviations: FDG, fluorodeoxy glucose 18; LD, largest diameter of lesion; PET, positron emission tomography.
[a] Standard uptake value of 18-FDG on PET scan.

observed in two patients (10.5%), partial response in 10 (53%), and stable disease in 5 (26%). Early progression occurred in two patients (10.5%). During follow-up, local progression occurred in eight nodules (42%) and the median time to progression was 27 months. There was no procedure-related mortality, although six deaths occurred during follow-up. The median follow-up in the remaining patients was 23 months. The probability of survival at 1 year was estimated to be 95% (95% confidence interval [CI], 0.68–0.91), and the median survival was not reached.

Stereotactic radiosurgery

Techniques

Radiation therapy is commonly used when resection for NSCLC is not possible. Five-year survival rates are usually poor, however, and have been reported from 10% to 30% [21–24]. Qiao and associates [24] summarized results from 18 studies reporting external beam radiation for stage I NSCLC. The mean 3- and 5-year survivals were 34% and 21%, respectively. Local tumor progression has been shown to be a major cause of failure after external beam radiation [21]. This can occur in up to 53% of patients [4]. Higher radiation doses seem to enhance local tumor control [25]. In one study, patients receiving greater than 70 Gy had better local control and cancer-specific survival than those treated with lower doses [26].

Increased doses of radiation, however, result in increased toxicity and damage to the surrounding pulmonary parenchyma, limiting dose escalation. The major toxicity encountered in treatment of lung tumors is pulmonary toxicity [27]. Radiation fibrosis seems to depend on the volume of lung radiated above a threshold of 20 to 30 Gy [27]. SRS is a relatively new approach that enables the selective delivery of an intense dose of high-energy radiation to destroy a tumor with precision targeting. The improved accuracy is achieved by very precise spatial localization of the tumor and delivery of multiple cross-fired beams of radiation to converge on the tumor, minimizing injury to surrounding normal tissue. This technology has become standard treatment in many centers for intracranial tumors (gamma knife). Unlike the brain, respiratory motion creates difficulties for the precise delivery of radiation to lung tumors. These respiratory displacements are greatest near the diaphragm and are less significant near the lung apex and adjacent to the carina. Only relatively recently have techniques become available that minimize the effects of respiratory motion on radiation delivery. One approach to SRS is to use breath-holding techniques, sometimes in combination with an abdominal compression device, to limit the ability of the diaphragm to move caudally [28].

The Cyberknife Stereotactic Radiosurgery System (Accuray, Sunnyvale, California) is a frameless SRS system that has been used in the University of Pittsburgh [29]. The Cyberknife System consists of a linear accelerator radiation source that is mounted on a robotic arm (Fig. 4). Before initiating treatment, two to four

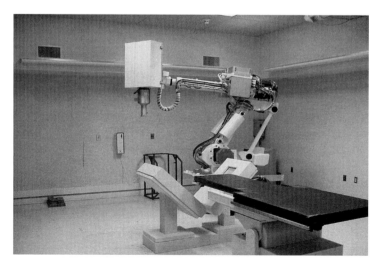

Fig. 4. Cyberknife system.

small gold fiducials (Fig. 5) are percutaneously placed close to the tumor using CT guidance. Recently, bronchoscopic deployment has become available under fluoroscopic guidance for central tumors. At the time of therapy, cameras on the Cyberknife System use these markers to localize the tumor in space. With the addition of the Synchrony option, breathing movements of a patient's chest are monitored and combined with real-time radiographic tracking of the fiducials to coordinate delivery of radiation during any point in the respiratory cycle. A major advantage with this system over those involving breath-holding and immobilization techniques is that the treatment times are shorter and better tolerated by patients (who usually have some degree of cardiopulmonary compromise).

Patient selection

Patient selection is virtually identical to that for RFA. An advantage of SRS, however, is that centrally based tumors can be treated. Additionally, the authors have found that some osteosarcomas are extremely difficult to penetrate with a needle, which is required for RFA. With SRS, fiducials need only to be positioned close to a tumor, rather than in a tumor. In the case of metastatic osteosarcoma, SRS may be the preferred ablation modality.

Results

Whyte and coworkers [30] published the first results of SRS for the lung using the Cyberknife

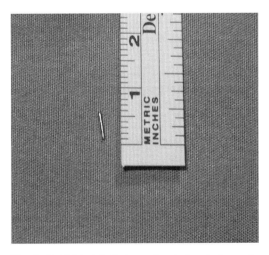

Fig. 5. Gold fiducials that are placed close to tumor to facilitate SRS.

System. This study included 23 patients from two institutions. Respiratory-gating was used in 14 patients and breath-holding in nine patients. A single fraction of 15 Gy was used. Three patients developed a pneumothorax following fiducial placement. There was no radiation esophagitis or clinically apparent radiation pneumonitis. At a mean follow-up of 7 months, two patients (8.6%) had a complete response; 15 (65.2%) a partial response; four (17.4%) had stable disease; and two (8.7%) had evidence of progression.

In the authors' initial experience at the University of Pittsburgh, 32 patients (27 with NSCLC and five with pulmonary metastases) were treated with SRS using the Cyberknife System [29]. Patients were treated with 20 Gy in a single fraction. It should be noted that the radiobiology of SRS (by virtue of a high single focused dose) is different from external beam radiation. The biologically effective dose is much higher [31]. It has been shown that higher biologically effective doses improve local progression-free survival [28,32]. In the authors' study, the 20-Gy dose was equivalent to a biologically effective dose of 60 to 70 Gy with standard techniques [29]. Following SRS in the 32 patients, an initial complete response was seen in seven (22%); partial response in 10 (31%); stable disease in nine (28%); and progression in five (16%). The probability of 1-year overall survival for the entire group and stage I patients was 78% (95% CI, 65–0.94) and 91% (95% CI, 75–1), respectively.

Both these studies demonstrate the safety and feasibility of SRS; however, results are still inferior to pulmonary resection. One question that is being investigated is whether increasing the SRS dose improves outcomes. Timmerman and colleagues [28] have previously reported the results of a dose escalation study in 37 patients with stage I NSCLC. A breath-holding technique with abdominal compression was used. In this series the dose was escalated from 20 to 60 Gy in three fractions. Complete response was seen in 27% of patients, and a partial response in 60%. At a median follow-up of 15 months, six patients (16.2%) had experienced local failure. All six received lower than 18 Gy, supporting the concept of dose escalation. The same group recently published a follow-up study [33]. Stage I NSCLC patients were stratified into T1 [19] and T2 [29] tumors. Dose-limiting toxicity included bronchitis, pericardial effusion, hypoxia, and pneumonitis. Local failure occurred in four (21%) of the T1 tumors and six

(21%) of the T2 tumors. In the T1 tumors, eight (42%) patients had regional or distant recurrences (or both). In the T2 tumors, six (21%) had regional or distant recurrence.

Longer follow-up and standardization of response criteria is needed to define better the value of SRS. The issue of optimal radiation dose also needs to be determined. Currently, a multicenter dose escalation study using the Cyberknife System with respiratory gating in all patients is being performed and it is hoped will address some of these issues.

Radiofrequency ablation and stereotactic radiosurgery

Each of the previously mentioned modalities (RFA and Cyberknife SRS) has its own benefits and limitations. In general, larger lesions have less desirable response with both of these techniques. Recently, the authors have been placing fiducial markers during RFA for larger lesions or asymmetric lesions where a uniform ablation could not be achieved. During the follow-up, if persistent tumor is suspected, it can be either treated with redo-RFA or SRS. Cyberknife SRS is more effective in this situation because the lesion is typically smaller in size as compared with the original lesion, because of the effect of RFA treatment.

Microwave ablation

MWA uses radiation in the 900 to 2450 MHz electromagnetic spectrum, resulting in dielectric heating (frictional heating of water molecules in tissue). As microwave radiation interacts with water molecules, the polarity of these molecules changes resulting in heating, eventually leading to cell death [34,35].

As with RFA, most clinical experience with MWA has been in the liver [36,37]. Unlike RFA, MWA is not limited by tissue boiling and charring of the tissue. This may allow temperatures within the targeted lesions to be driven higher, resulting in a larger ablation zone in a shorter period of time. MWA has been compared with RFA (using the RITA system) in a hepatic porcine model in 19 pigs. The pigs were sacrificed at 0, 2, and 28 days after ablation. To assess the heat-sink effect of blood vessels on ablation the investigators created a deflection score. This was defined by measuring the diameter of the zone of ablation at a blood

vessel (>3 mm) and the diameter of the ablation zone next to the same blood vessel. The percentage difference between these diameters was the deflection score. The deflection score was significantly less ($P < .02$) after MVA (3.6%) compared with RFA (17%). The ablation zone was significantly ($P < .01$) greater in the long axis after MWA (3.6 cm) compared with RFA (2.2 cm). There were no differences, however, in short axis measurement or tumor volume. The differences in length of ablation may have been related to the protocol design in that for MVA a 3.6-cm electrode was used, whereas for RFA only a 3-cm deployment of the RITA probe was performed.

Shibata and associates [36] performed a randomized comparison of MVA (N = 36) and RFA (N = 36) for small hepatocellular carcinomas. There were no significant differences noted in the rates of initial therapeutic effect, complications, and residual disease.

Clinical experience with MWA for lung is limited at this time. Feng and coworkers [38] reported on the MWA of 28 tumors in 20 patients. A response of 50% or more was noted in 13 (46.4%) of the nodules and a complete response in three (10.7%). No significant complications were noted. An ablate and resect study was performed by Simon and coauthors [35]. Patients undergoing elective lung resection underwent MWA before resection. The mean tumor diameter was 3 cm (range, 2–5.5 cm), with an average tumor volume of 7.1 cm³. The maximum ablation achieved was 4 cm (3–5 cm), with a tumor volume of 23.4 cm³. Further experience with this modality is necessary before the role of MWA can be established in the treatment of early stage lung cancer.

The politics and controversies of percutaneous ablation

With the advent of percutaneous ablation techniques for the treatment of early stage lung cancer, controversy has emerged regarding the optimal approach in treating these patients. These controversial issues are being driven by the emergence of exciting new technology, aggressive interventional radiologists motivated at implementing these techniques into their practice, the patient's natural tendency to seek out less invasive interventions, and the earlier detection of smaller, more easily treatable lesions.

A primary issue relates to who should be doing these procedures: experienced interventional radiologists with surgical "back-up," surgeons with extensive experience in minimally invasive and percutaneous CT-guided techniques, or a combined approach whereby the radiologist performs a lung biopsy and the surgeon performs the RFA. A variety of scenarios have occurred at different centers, based on institutional and departmental biases, and the available expertise and interest of the surgical and radiology staff. A similar procedural evolution occurred with the implementation of video-assisted thorascopic surgery techniques. The Society of Thoracic Surgeons/American Association for Thoracic Surgery Position Statement on video-assisted thorascopic surgery has recommended that such procedures be performed by surgeons familiar with open thoracic surgical approaches and the management of their complications. The surgeon must have the judgment, training, and capability to proceed to an open thoracic procedure if necessary, and should personally guide the preoperative and postoperative care of the patient [39]. Although aggressive interventional radiology technicians may have the experience and ability to perform difficult percutaneous interventions, there is great variability in their clinical training, and many may have never studied or treated patients with lung cancer. Conversely, many thoracic surgeons have dedicated their entire training and career to treating lung cancer, and perform minimally invasive and percutaneous procedures on a daily basis. Thoracic surgeons are specifically trained in the areas of pulmonary physiology and oncology, are personally capable of managing procedure-related complications, are involved in the primary and follow-up care of patients with cancer, and have developed a historical association with consultants in the management of this disease. There is no doubt, however, that complacency of thoracic surgical leadership can lead to a critical deficiency in embracing and incorporating these new techniques in a timely manner, resulting in a loss of control of these modalities and potentially the patients themselves.

Credentialing is also an important and controversial issue. Hospital administration and departmental guidelines have to be established to identify those physicians approved to conduct these procedures. Surgeons need to complete a dedicated didactic session covering the basic knowledge-base and techniques, in conjunction with a period of proctorship until proficiency is demonstrated after performing a prescribed number of CT-guided interventions. Currently, there are no nationally accepted standards for the credentialing of surgeons to perform RFA within the chest. Gaining access to a CT scanner can also be a complicated process. Operating rooms with a built-in CT scanner offer the ideal environment for performing these procedures. The necessary surgical equipment and staff are on hand, making the procedure safer and more efficient. If the procedures must be performed in the radiology suite, negotiations must be performed regarding establishing a block time to schedule cases. The room must be capable of supporting an anesthesia circuit, with built-in oxygen and suction. All supplies related to the procedure must be stored on-site, or in a portable cart. Quality assurance programs must be implemented to ensure optimal patient outcomes, with a database monitoring patient morbidity and mortality profiles.

Thoracic surgeons are best suited to make the decision as to which surgical or ablative modality to use in any given clinical setting. Whether to use an open, thoracoscopic, or percutaneous technique to manage a patient with a small pulmonary nodule requires careful judgment and expertise with each technique to ensure an optimal oncologic outcome. Certainly, percutaneous therapeutic modalities will ultimately have a role in high-risk patients with compromised lung function. Decision-making can be even more complex in managing patients with difficult lesions, such as ground-glass opacities (see the article by Yoshida elsewhere in this issue). These lesions tend to be small, slow-growing, and have a more indolent natural history. Many of these lesions may represent carcinoma in situ or minimally invasive cancers where anatomic resection with or without lymph node dissection may not be necessary [40]. The use of percutaneous ablative techniques in this setting may represent an ideal application of this technology.

As these innovative techniques are developed and refined, careful attention must be paid to several important pitfalls including overapplication of these modalities in the setting of indeterminate solitary pulmonary nodules, inappropriate or inadequate management of small to medium sized lung cancer, inappropriate interventions directed toward metastatic disease, and the risk of inadequately staging patients before intervention. To avoid these pitfalls, thoracic surgeons should maintain a leadership position in the deployment of these techniques for the treatment of patients with thoracic malignancies.

Summary

RFA and SRS have been demonstrated to be safe with reasonable efficacy in the treatment of small lung tumors. It is unclear which option is the most effective in the treatment of NSCLC, with both RFA and SRS demonstrating similar early response and progression rates. RFA can be performed in one treatment session, whereas it now seems that SRS is more effective if larger doses of radiation over two to three fractions are performed. RFA is not recommended for centrally based tumors. There are also some tumors (eg, small apical tumors, posteriorly positioned tumors close to the diaphragm, and tumors close to the scapula) where it may be difficult percutaneously to position an active electrode. Such patients are more optimally treated with SRS. In certain circumstances, a combined approach may be beneficial (RFA and SRS).

At this point in time, MWA is the least well developed modality. Although treatment times and heat-sink effect may be less compared with RFA, larger trials are needed to understand better the impact of this factor on effectiveness and safety. The heat-sink effect may be protective, minimizing the necrosis of large blood vessels and the risk of subsequent fatal hemoptysis.

Future studies need to address long-term outcomes using standardized assessments of treatment response between centers. Comparisons between different RFA systems and ablation modalities need to be undertaken to delineate the optimal use of these strategies in the treatment of early stage lung cancer. Until long-term data with these ablative techniques become available, surgical resection should be performed when clinically possible.

References

[1] Jemal A, Siegel R, Ward E, et al. Cancer statistics, 2006. CA Cancer J Clin 2006;56:106–30.

[2] Bach PB, Cramer LD, Warren JL, et al. Racial differences in the treatment of early stage non-small cell lung cancer. N Engl J Med 1999;341:1198–205.

[3] Kupelian PA, Komaki R, Allen P. Prognostic factors in the treatment of node-negative non-small cell lung carcinoma with radiation alone. Int J Radiat Oncol Biol Phys 1996;36:607–13.

[4] Zierhut D, Bettscheider C, Schubert K, et al. Radiation therapy of stage I and II non-small cell lung cancer. Lung Cancer 2001;34:S39–43.

[5] Sutherland LM, Williams JA, Padbury RT, et al. Radiofrequency ablation of liver tumors: a systematic review. Arch Surg 2006;141(2):181–90.

[6] Jungraithmayr W, Burger D, Olschewski M, et al. Cryoablation of malignant liver tumors: results of a single center study. Hepatobiliary Pancreat Dis Int 2005;4(4):554–60.

[7] Livraghi T, Solbiati L, Meloni MF, et al. Treatment of focal liver tumors with percutaneous radio-frequency ablation: complications encountered in a multicenter study. Radiology 2003;226:441–51.

[8] Dupuy DE, Zagoria RJ, Akerley W, et al. Percutaneous radiofrequency ablation of malignancies in the lung. AJR Am J Roentgenol 2000;174(1):57–9.

[9] Schaefer O, Lohrman C, Langer M. CT guided radiofrequency ablation of a bronchogenic carcinoma. Br J Radiol 2003;76:268–70.

[10] Goldberg SN, Gazelle GS, Compton CC, et al. Radiofrequency tissue ablation of VX2 tumor nodules in the rabbit lung. Acad Radiol 1996;3:929–35.

[11] Miao Y, Ni Y, Bosmans H, et al. Radiofrequency ablation for eradication of pulmonary tumor in rabbits. J Surg Res 2001;99:265–71.

[12] Yang S, Whyte R, Askin F, et al. Radiofrequency ablation of primary and metastatic lung tumors: analysis of an ablate and resect study. Presented at the American Association for Thoracic Surgery 82nd Annual Meeting. Washington, DC, May 5–8, 2002.

[13] Nguyen CL, Scott WJ, Young NA, et al. Radiofrequency ablation of primary lung cancer: results from an ablate and resect pilot study. Chest 2005;128:3507–11.

[14] Denys AL, De Baere T, Kuoch V, et al. Radiofrequency tissue ablation of the liver in vivo and ex vivo experiments with four different systems. Eur Radiol 2003;13:2346–52.

[15] Battafarano RJ, Meyers BF, Guthrie TJ, et al. Surgical resection of multifocal non-small cell lung cancer is associated with prolonged survival. Ann Thorac Surg 2002;74:988–93.

[16] Herrera LJ, Fernando HC, Perry Y, et al. Radiofrequency ablation of pulmonary malignant tumors in non-surgical candidates. J Thorac Cardiovasc Surg 2003;125:29–937.

[17] Suh RD, Wallace AB, Sheehan RE, et al. Unresectable pulmonary malignancies: CT guided percutaneous radiofrequency ablation. Preliminary results. Radiology 2003;229:821–9.

[18] Fernando HC, De Hoyos A, Landreneau RJ, et al. Radiofrequency ablation for the treatment of non-small cell lung cancer in marginal surgical candidates. J Thorac Cardiovasc Surg 2005;129:261–7.

[19] Steinke K, Sewell PE, Dupuy D, et al. Pulmonary radiofrequency ablation: an international study survey. Anticancer Res 2004;24:339–43.

[20] Pennathur A, Luketich JD, Abbas G, et al. Radiofrequency abalation for treatment of stage I non-small cell lung cancer in high-risk patients. J Thorac Cardiovasc Surg 2007, in press.

[21] Jeremic B, Classen J, Bamberg M. Radiotherapy alone for medically inoperable, early stage (I/II) non-small cell lung cancer. Int J Radiat Oncol Biol Phys 2002;54:119–30.

[22] Sibley G, Jaimeson T, Marks L, et al. Radiotherapy alone for stage I non-small cell lung cancer: the Duke experience. Int J Radiat Oncol Biol Phys 1998;40: 149–54.

[23] Kaskowitz L, Graham MV, Emani B, et al. Radiation therapy alone for stage I non-small cell lung cancer. Int J Radiat Oncol Biol Phys 1993;27: 517–23.

[24] Qiao X, Tullgren O, Lax I, et al. The role of radiotherapy in treatment of stage I non-small cell lung cancer. Lung Cancer 2003;41:1–11.

[25] Bauermann M, Appold S, Peterson S, et al. Dose and fractionation concepts in the primary radiotherapy of non-small cell lung cancer. Lung Cancer 2001; 33(Suppl):S35–45.

[26] Bradley JD, Ieumwananonthachai N, Purdy JA, et al. Gross tumor volume, critical prognostic factor in patients with three-dimensional conformal radiation therapy for non-small cell lung cancer. Int J Radiat Oncol Biol Phys 2002;52(1):49–57.

[27] Abratt RP, Morgan GW. Lung toxicity following chest irradiation in patients with lung cancer. Lung Cancer 2002;35(2):103–9.

[28] Timmerman R, Papiez L, McGarry R, et al. Extracranial stereotactic radioablation: results of a phase I study in medically inoperable stage I non-small cell lung cancer. Chest 2003;124:1946–55.

[29] Pennathur A, Luketich JD, Burton S, et al. Stereotactic radiosurgery for the treatment of lung neoplasm: initial experience. Ann Thorac Surg 2007; 83:1820–5.

[30] Whyte RI, Crownover R, Murphy MJ, et al. Stereotactic radiosurgery for lung tumors: preliminary report of a phase I trial. Ann Thorac Surg 2003;75: 1097–101.

[31] Timmerman RD, Papiez L. The Song/Kavanagh/Benedcict et al. Article reviewed. Oncology 2004; 18:1430–5.

[32] Martel M, Ten Haken R, Hazuka M, et al. Estimation of tumor control probability from 3-D dose distributions of non-small cell lung cancer patients. Lung Cancer 1999;24:31–7.

[33] McGarry RC, Papiez L, Williams M, et al. Stereotactic body radiation therapy of early-stage non-small cell lung carcinoma: phase I study. Int J Radiat Oncol Biol Phys 2005;63:1010–5.

[34] Furukawa K, Toyoaki M, Kato Y, et al. Microwave coagulation therapy in canine peripheral lung tissue. J Surg Res 2005;123:245–50.

[35] Simon CS, Dupuy DE, Mayo-Smith WW. Microwave ablation: principles and applications. Radiographics 2005;25:S69–83.

[36] Shibata T, Iimuro Y, Yammoto Y, et al. Small hepatocellular carcinoma; comparison of radiofrequency ablation and percutaneous microwave coagulation therapy. Radiology 2002;223:331–7.

[37] Lu MD, Chen JW, Xie XY, et al. Hepatocellular carcinoma: US-guided percutaneous microwave coagulation therapy. Radiology 2001;221:167–72.

[38] Feng W, Liu W, Liu C, et al. Percutaneous microwave coagulation therapy for lung cancer. Zhonghua Zhong Liu Za Zhi 2002;24:388–90.

[39] McNeally MF, Lewis RJ, Anderson RJ, et al. Statement of the STS/AATS joint committee on thoracoscopy and video-assisted thoracic surgery. J Thorac Cardiovasc Surg 1992;104(1):1.

[40] Noguchi M, Morikawa A, Kawasaki M, et al. Small adenocarcinoma of the lung: histologic characteristics and prognosis. Cancer 1995;75(12): 2844–52.

THORACIC
SURGERY
CLINICS

Thorac Surg Clin 17 (2007) 273–278

Role of Adjuvant Radiation (External Beam/Brachytherapy) for Stage I NSCLC

Ara Ketchedjian, MD[a], Thomas A. DiPetrillo, MD[b],
Benedict Daly, MD[a], Hiran C. Fernando, MBBS, FRCS[a],*

[a]Department of Cardiothoracic Surgery, Boston Medical Center, 88 East Newton Street,
Robinson B-402, Boston, MA 02118–2392, USA
[b]Department of Radiation Oncology, Brown Medical School, Rhode Island Hospital,
593 Eddy Street, Providence, RI 02903, USA

In 1995, the Lung Cancer Study Group published the results of the only randomized study comparing sublobar resection and lobectomy [1]. The principal finding in this study was a threefold increase in local recurrence from 6.4% to 17.2% in patients having sublobar resection. At follow-up that extended to 72 months, there was only a trend ($P = .088$) favoring better survival in the lobectomy patients. Since the publication of this study, lobectomy alone has remained the standard of care for stage I non–small cell lung cancer (NSCLC). Following the results of several randomized trials [2–5], it has become standard to use adjuvant chemotherapy for resected stages Ib, II, and III NSCLC. More recently, a follow-up study of the patients in one of these trials demonstrated that the survival advantage initially seen for stage Ib NSCLC did not hold true with longer follow-up, bringing into question again the role of adjuvant chemotherapy for stage Ib cancers [5].

This article reviews the role of adjuvant radiation following surgical treatment of NSCLC. Currently, radiation is not routinely used following lobar resection for NSCLC, although there may be a role following lesser resections or ablation of NSCLC [6,7]. Radiation therapy despite its benefits is associated with cellular toxicity, potentially adding to treatment morbidity. After lung resection for NSCLC, adjuvant treatment with radiation may injure surrounding normal tissue resulting in pulmonary, cardiac, esophageal, or musculoskeletal complications. In patients with impaired pulmonary function this represents a significant morbidity. Monson and colleagues [8] looked at patients receiving radiotherapy as adjuvant and definitive therapy and noted an almost 20% incidence of pneumonitis. Advocates of adjuvant radiotherapy cite improved technologies and techniques that allow the administration of radiation without a higher incidence of morbidity [9].

The role of radiation after complete resection of non–small cell lung cancer

The largest study looking at postoperative radiation therapy following the surgical resection of NSCLC was a meta-analysis published by the Postoperative Radiation Therapy (PORT) Meta-Analysis Trialists Group [10]. The PORT study included 2128 patients from nine separate randomized trials and compared observation versus adjuvant radiotherapy following surgical resection. It should be emphasized that this study did not differentiate between patients undergoing lobectomy and those undergoing sublobar resections, although the authors' mentioned that only trials where complete resection was performed were included in the analysis. At a median follow-up of 3.9 years there was a 21% relative

* Corresponding author.
E-mail address: hiran.fernando@bmc.org
(H.C. Fernando).

increase in the risk of death in patients treated with adjuvant radiotherapy. Although a 24% reduction in the risk of local recurrence when radiation was used was seen, this benefit was countered by the adverse effect that radiation had on survival. Local recurrence-free survival was worse following radiation. Subgroup analysis demonstrated that the adverse effect on survival was present for those patients with stage I to II, but not for stage III patients with N2 disease. Other studies have demonstrated a similar increase in mortality following adjuvant radiotherapy. Dautzenberg and colleagues [11] compared irradiated stage I to III NSCLC with surgery alone and found no significant difference in local recurrence or metastatic disease. There was, however, an increase in the rate of noncancer deaths seemingly related to dose per fraction delivered.

Since the publication of the PORT analysis their results have been scrutinized and debated. Major points of contention among proponents of radiotherapy have been focused on the technology and techniques of radiotherapy delivery. The source of radiation energy used, within a number of trials included in the PORT analysis, is of concern. Many patients were treated with older radiotherapy sources, such as cobalt 60, which by current standards is believed to be substandard. Toxicity has also proved to be related to radiation dose (both total and fractional) and volume of normal tissue included in the radiation fields. Introduction of newer modalities for the planning and delivery of radiotherapy and practical, biologically appropriate fractionation schema has helped to reduce the exposure of healthy tissues and reduce the observed detrimental effects of external beam radiation following surgical resection.

A small handful of trials have begun to look at adjuvant radiation following the resection of early stage lung cancer. One such recent randomized trial of stage I NSCLC patients was reported by Trodella and colleagues [12]. In this study, 104 stage Ia and Ib patients were randomized to no therapy or adjuvant radiation following lobar resection for NSCLC. The adjuvant radiotherapy was given using relatively modern techniques. The radiation arm demonstrated fewer local recurrences (2.2% versus 23%). Disease-free survival (71% versus 60%; $P = .039$) and overall survival (67% versus 58%; $P = .048$) were better in the radiation group. Six patients (11.7%) experienced a grade 1 acute toxicity, and 19 (37.3%) patients developed postradiation pulmonary fibrosis. Although these results might favor a re-examination of the role of radiation following resection of early stage NSCLC, the local recurrence rate of 23% in the surgery-only group is much higher than what is normally reported for NSCLC after lobectomy. At the present time, the authors do not believe that there is a role for radiation therapy following lobar resection for stage I NSCLC.

Role of radiation following sublobar resection

Currently, sublobar resection is considered a compromise procedure that is reserved for those patients who are believed to be at increased risk from a lobar resection. Locoregional failure has been the Achilles heel of limited pulmonary resection.

One mode of failure for resected early stage tumors can be attributed to residual tumor cells. Goldstein and colleagues [13] assessed T1N0 peripheral adenocarcinomas treated by wedge resection followed by lobectomy. Residual adenocarcinoma was found in 45% of the completion lobectomy specimens. The mean microscopic margin was 0.7 mm in these patients with residual disease compared with 2.4 mm in those without. In this study, all patients underwent planned lobectomy. Generally, most surgeons strive to achieve wider margins when using sublobar resection as the only intended resection for NSCLC. Patient factors, however, such as the ability to tolerate single lung ventilation during the procedure, and the location of the tumor within the lobe, may impair the ability to achieve a good margin. The impact of margin size was analyzed in 81 patients with stage I NSCLC treated with intended sublobar resection because of pulmonary compromise [14]. Local recurrence was significantly ($P = .04$) lower when the margin of resection was 1 cm or more (7.5% versus 14.6%).

Gross margins frequently underestimate the microscopic margin. Different methods have been used to evaluate histologic margins following limited resection. Sawabata and colleagues [15] used slides brushed along the staple-line to evaluate histologic positivity following resection. Their methodology revealed a 47% positive rate for residual malignant cells. Those patients with cytologically positive cells demonstrated a 57% margin relapse rate compared with 0% among those with negative cytologic margins.

The significance of these findings demonstrates the potential need for adjuvant treatment following sublobar resection of stage I tumors.

Analogous to the evolving treatment of breast cancer, limited resection surgery with adjuvant radiation may yield similar oncologic results to lobar resection while conserving functional capacity.

This is not a new idea. Miller and Hatcher [16] reported their experience with sublobar resection for patients with impaired pulmonary function. In their study, 32 patients underwent wedge or segmental resection. Adjuvant radiation was used in 18 patients in a cone-down fashion to the area of the primary lesion and the hilum. Local recurrence was much lower in the patients receiving radiation therapy (6.25% versus 35%). More recently, the Cancer and Leukemia Group B performed a multicenter phase II prospective trial evaluating the feasibility of thoracoscopic wedge resection followed by local radiotherapy in high-risk patients with clinical T1 lesions [17]. Radiation consisted of 56 Gy delivered to the staple line with a 2-cm margin. Of 65 patients who were accrued, 58 were eligible. Video-assisted thoracic surgery resection was successfully performed in 79% of pathologic T1 lesions and 50% of pathologic T2 lesions. A margin of 1 cm or more was only achieved in 46% of the patients. Only 32 patients were found to have pathologically staged T1 lesions. Of these patients, three refused radiotherapy and one died before starting radiotherapy. Pneumonitis occurred in 4% and severe dyspnea was reported in 11% of these 28 patients. This study illustrates the difficulty with delivering adjuvant radiation to a population of patients that are already compromised with respect to their pulmonary function. Any additional injury from radiation can be seriously problematic. Also, postoperative patients may be reluctant to return to the hospital for their radiation treatments. This was seen in this study, where 9.4% of eligible patients refused their protocol radiation therapy.

Some centers are using adjuvant brachytherapy to compensate for the difficulties associated with postoperative external beam treatment [6]. Brachytherapy uses radioactive seeds that can be placed along the resected margin at the time of lung resection. The advantage of intraoperative brachytherapy is that this provides a mean of delivering radiation in a more uniform manner to the staple line area, with a 100% patient compliance. As seen in the previously mentioned studies, an adequate resection margin is frequently not achieved, particularly when a compromised (nonlobar) resection is used for a compromised patient. The chance of local failure is increased in these patients, and the addition of brachytherapy theoretically should minimize this occurrence.

Two techniques have been described in the use of brachytherapy following limited resection. The first technique involves the placement of paired sutures placed adjacent to the staple lines [18]. These sutures contain iodine-125 seeds that deliver the radiation. The sutures are a commercially available product (Amersham Health, Princeton, New Jersey). The second technique involves placement of the same sutures into a vicryl mesh that is then placed over the staple line [6]. Typically, about four parallel suture strands are placed in the mesh to deliver a dose of 10,000 to 12,000 cGy to the resection margin to a 0.5-cm depth. One study reported the use of brachytherapy using the paired suture technique in 33 high-risk patients, primarily after wedge resection. The local recurrence rate was 6.1%, which was similar to the 6.4% reported after lobectomy in the Lung Cancer Study Group study. There were no patients who developed pneumonitis. A retrospective study from Pittsburgh compared local recurrence rates in 98 patients undergoing sublobar resection with brachytherapy with 102 patients undergoing sublobar resection alone [19]. There was no difference in operative mortality, distal recurrence, or survival. Local recurrence was significantly reduced, however, from 18.6% to 2% in those patients who had adjuvant brachytherapy. In comparison with the study using the paired suture technique, most operations were segmentectomy rather than wedge resections. As in the earlier study, there was no incidence of pneumonitis in patients treated with adjuvant brachytherapy. In a more recent multicenter retrospective study looking at stage 1A cancers, brachytherapy was used in 60 of 124 sublobar resections. Local recurrence was significantly lower in those patients who had brachytherapy at 3.3% compared with 17.2% for those patients treated with sublobar resection alone [20]. Birdas and colleagues [21] compared 41 stage Ib patients treated with sublobar resection and brachytherapy with 126 stage Ib patients treated with lobectomy. Local recurrence was similar (3.2% versus 4.8%) in the two groups. Despite significantly greater impairment of pulmonary function in the sublobar group, 4-year survival was similar (54.1% versus 51.8%).

The preliminary results of sublobar resection with adjuvant brachytherapy are promising. Currently, the American College of Surgeons

Oncology Group is performing a multicenter randomized trial in patients with T1N0 cancers, in patients who are believed to be at increased risk for lobectomy. After the decision to perform sublobar resection has been made patients are randomized to either sublobar resection alone or sublobar resection with brachytherapy. One concern that has arisen as sites have introduced this technique to their centers is the radiation risk to staff. The group from Pittsburgh recently reported on a series of 10 patients undergoing brachytherapy with mesh implants [22]. Microdosimeters were placed on the back of each hand of the surgeon and radiation oncologist during these procedures. Patients had 40 to 60 seeds implanted with a median total activity of 23.6 mCi. In contrast, the median dose to the physicians' was minimal at 2 mrem, demonstrating that this is a safe technique for treating lung cancer with respect to health care professionals.

Adjuvant radiation following radiofrequency ablation of lung cancers

Radiofrequency ablation (RFA) is a relatively new modality that has been used to treat patients with lung tumors who are believed to be at too high-risk to undergo any resection [23–25]. Long-term outcomes are not yet available; however, intermediate outcomes are increasingly being reported. The use of RFA was recently reported in a group of high-risk patients with NSCLC treated with RFA [26]. Within this group, nine patients had stage I disease. The mean progression-free interval was 17.6 months, with 35% of patients demonstrating local progression. A follow-up study involving 19 stage I patients was recently reported [27]. At a median follow-up of 27 months, local progression was seen in 42% of patients. As with sublobar resection, one possible way to combat this high local recurrence is with adjuvant radiation. Hypoxic cells tend to be resistant to radiation, and the central areas of tumors are relatively hypoxic. RFA is more effective in the more dense central areas of a cancer. RFA also induces a surrounding area of inflammation with neovascularization. Following RFA, radiation may be more effective in treating the periphery of a tumor [7]. This concept was investigated in a rat tumor model [28]. Rats were divided into groups that received no treatment, radiation alone, RFA alone, or RFA and radiation. In the control group median survival was 12 days. In the RFA or radiation alone this was 20 days. In the group

receiving RFA and radiation median survival was 120 days. Dupuy and colleagues [7] recently reported on 24 stage I patients treated with RFA followed by three-dimensional conformal radiation therapy to a dose of 66 Gy. In this series there was more than 90% local control (2 of 24 local recurrences), although 9 of 24 patients experienced systemic recurrence. At a mean follow-up of 26.7 months, 2- and 5-year survivals were 50% and 39%, respectively. Out of 14 deaths, three (21.4%) were deemed respiratory in nature. No patients experienced acute radiation pneumonitis clinically and two patients were believed to have significant delayed parenchymal fibrosis on CT scans without associated respiratory symptoms. These data are interesting and support further investigation of combining RFA with radiation. Because patients treated with RFA are impaired with respect to their pulmonary function, the addition of external beam radiation may lead to further deterioration in lung function. Certainly, this may have contributed in part to the three deaths from respiratory failure. Future investigation should focus on alternative methods of radiation, such as stereotactic radiosurgery [29].

Summary

There seems to be no role for adjuvant radiation in stage I NSCLC patients treated by lobectomy. Adjuvant brachytherapy in combination with sublobar resection is a promising approach that seems to decrease local recurrence rates similar to that reported following lobectomy. If the results of the current American College of Surgeons Oncology Group randomized trial are favorable, it may be possible in the future to define subgroups of patients with stage I NSCLC who are able to be treated with this approach in preference to lobectomy. Until further data are available, lobectomy should remain the standard of care. RFA is an alternative for the high-risk patient with NSCLC who is considered too high-risk even for sublobar resection. Although long-term results are not yet available, it does seem that local recurrence is a significant problem. In a similar fashion to the approach currently being investigated with sublobar resection, the addition of radiation may improve local control after RFA. In particular, adjuvant stereotactic radiation should be investigated as a potential method of decreasing local recurrence and preserving lung function in these high-risk patients.

References

[1] Ginsberg RJ, Rubinstein LV. Lung Cancer Study Group. Randomized trial of lobectomy versus limited resection for T1 N0 non-small cell lung cancer. Ann Thorac Surg 1995;60(3):615–22 [discussion: 622–13].

[2] Winton T, Livingston R, Johnson D, et al. Vinorelbine plus cisplatin vs. observation in resected non-small-cell lung cancer. N Engl J Med 2005;352(25): 2589–97.

[3] Douillard J, Delena M, et al. ANITA: phase III adjuvant vinorelbine and cisplatin versus observation in completely resected (stage I-III) non-small cell lung cancer patients: final results after 70-month median follow-up. J Clin Oncol 2005;(Suppl 16S):624S.

[4] Strauss GM, Maddaus MA, et al. Randomized clinical trial of adjuvant chemotherapy with paclitaxel and carboplatin following resection in stage IB non-small cell lung cancer (NSCLC): report of Cancer and Leukemia Group B (CALGB) Protocol 9633. Proceedings of the American Society of Clinical Oncology 2004; abstract7019.

[5] Arriagada R, Bergman B, Dunant A, et al. Cisplatin-based adjuvant chemotherapy in patients with completely resected non-small-cell lung cancer. N Engl J Med 2004;350(4):351–60.

[6] d'Amato TA, Galloway M, Szydlowski G, et al. Intraoperative brachytherapy following thoracoscopic wedge resection of stage I lung cancer. Chest 1998;114(4):1112–5.

[7] Dupuy DE, DiPetrillo T, Gandhi S, et al. Radiofrequency ablation followed by conventional radiotherapy for medically inoperable stage I non-small cell lung cancer. Chest 2006;129(3):738–45.

[8] Monson JM, Stark P, Reilly JJ, et al. Clinical radiation pneumonitis and radiographic changes after thoracic radiation therapy for lung carcinoma. Cancer 1998;82(5):842–50.

[9] Bogart JA, Aronowitz JN. Localized non-small cell lung cancer: adjuvant radiotherapy in the era of effective systemic therapy. Clin Cancer Res 2005; 11(13 Pt 2):5004s–10s.

[10] PORT Meta-analysis Trialists Group. Postoperative radiotherapy in non-small-cell lung cancer: systematic review and meta-analysis of individual patient data from nine randomised controlled trials. Lancet 1998;352(9124):257–63.

[11] Dautzenberg B, Arriagada R, Chammard AB, et al. A controlled study of postoperative radiotherapy for patients with completely resected nonsmall cell lung carcinoma. Groupe d'Etude et de Traitement des Cancers Bronchiques. Cancer 1999;86(2): 265–73.

[12] Trodella L, Granone P, Valente S, et al. Adjuvant radiotherapy in non-small cell lung cancer with pathological stage I: definitive results of a phase III randomized trial. Radiother Oncol 2002;62(1): 11–9.

[13] Goldstein NS, Ferkowicz M, Kestin L, et al. Wedge resection margin distances and residual adenocarcinoma in lobectomy specimens. Am J Clin Pathol 2003;120(5):720–4.

[14] El-Sherif ASR, Fernando HC, Santos R, et al. Margin and local recurrence after resection of non-small cell lung cancer. Paper presented at the Society of Surgical Oncology. Atlanta (GA), March 3–6, 2005.

[15] Sawabata N, Matsumura A, Ohota M, et al. Cytologically malignant margins of wedge resected stage I non-small cell lung cancer. Ann Thorac Surg 2002; 74(6):1953–7.

[16] Miller JI, Hatcher CR Jr. Limited resection of bronchogenic carcinoma in the patient with marked impairment of pulmonary function. Ann Thorac Surg 1987;44(4):340–3.

[17] Shennib H, Bogart J, Herndon JE, et al. Video-assisted wedge resection and local radiotherapy for peripheral lung cancer in high-risk patients: the Cancer and Leukemia Group B (CALGB) 9335, a phase II, multi-institutional cooperative group study. J Thorac Cardiovasc Surg 2005; 129(4):813–8.

[18] Lee W, Daly BD, DiPetrillo TA, et al. Limited resection for non-small cell lung cancer: observed local control with implantation of I-125 brachytherapy seeds. Ann Thorac Surg 2003;75(1):237–42 [discussion: 242–33].

[19] Santos R, Colonias A, Parda D, et al. Comparison between sublobar resection and 125 iodine brachytherapy after sublobar resection in high-risk patients with stage I non-small-cell lung cancer. Surgery 2003;134(4):691–7 [discussion: 697].

[20] Fernando HC, Santos RS, Benfield JR, et al. Lobar and sublobar resection with and without brachytherapy for small stage IA non-small cell lung cancer. J Thorac Cardiovasc Surg 2005;129(2): 261–7.

[21] Birdas TJ, Koehler RP, Colonias A, et al. Sublobar resection with brachytherapy versus lobectomy for stage Ib nonsmall cell lung cancer. Ann Thorac Surg 2006;81(2):434–8 [discussion: 438–9].

[22] Smith R, Komanduri K, Burton S, et al. Dosimetric evaluation of physician and staff radiation exposure during I125 vicryl mesh implants. Paper presented at the RSNA2005 Connecting for Lifelong Learning. Chicago, November 27–December 3, 2005.

[23] Dupuy DE, Zagoria RJ, Akerley W, et al. Percutaneous radiofrequency ablation of malignancies in the lung. AJR Am J Roentgenol 2000;174(1): 57–9.

[24] Herrera LJ, Fernando HC, Perry Y, et al. Radiofrequency ablation of pulmonary malignant tumors in nonsurgical candidates. J Thorac Cardiovasc Surg 2003;125(4):929–37.

[25] Ketchedjian A, Daly B, Luketich J, et al. Minimally invasive techniques for managing pulmonary

metastases: video-assisted thoracic surgery and radiofrequency ablation. Thorac Surg Clin 2006; 16(2):157–65.

[26] Fernando HC, De Hoyos A, Landreneau RJ, et al. Radiofrequency ablation for the treatment of non-small cell lung cancer in marginal surgical candidates. J Thorac Cardiovasc Surg 2005;129(3):639–44.

[27] Pennathur A, Abbas G. Radiofrequency ablation for the treatment of stage I non-small cell lung cancer in high risk patients. Paper presented at the Western Thoracic Surgical Association Annual Meeting. Sun Valley (ID), June 21–24, 2006.

[28] Horkan C, Dalal K, Coderre JA, et al. Reduced tumor growth with combined radiofrequency ablation and radiation therapy in a rat breast tumor model. Radiology 2005;235(1):81–8.

[29] Whyte RI, Crownover R, Murphy MJ, et al. Stereotactic radiosurgery for lung tumors: preliminary report of a phase I trial. Ann Thorac Surg 2003; 75(4):1097–101.

ELSEVIER
SAUNDERS

Thorac Surg Clin 17 (2007) 279–285

THORACIC
SURGERY
CLINICS

Role of Adjuvant Systemic Therapy for Stage I NSCLC

Eric Vallières, MD, FRCSC

Lung Cancer Program, Swedish Cancer Institute, 1101 Madison Street,
Suite 850, Seattle, WA 98104, USA

Results of trials reported in the last 4 years have convincingly demonstrated a role for adjuvant or postoperative chemotherapy in the management of good performance status patients after a complete resection of their stages II and IIIA non–small cell lung carcinoma (NSCLC) [1–4]. The role of chemotherapy after surgery of stage I disease, however, remains a subject of debate. This article reviews the limited data that have evaluated this approach in early stage disease and set the stage for future trials in this population of patients.

Stage IA

None of the recent North American adjuvant chemotherapy trials have included patients with resected IA disease. In Europe, stage IA patients made up 10% of the patients in the International Adjuvant Lung cancer Trial (IALT) [1] and were also included in the Adjuvant Lung Project Italy trial (ALPI) [5]. They were, however, excluded from the Adjuvant Navelbine International Trialist Association trial (ANITA) (Table 1) [3]. In Japan, large studies have targeted these patients and these results are discussed separately.

The IALT trial randomized a total of 1867 patients after complete resection of stages I, II, and IIIA NSCLC to receive a cisplatin-based doublet or not after surgery. Only 10% of these subjects had stage IA disease. The absolute 5-year survival was increased by 4.1% (*P* < .03) for the whole population, but when allowing subset analysis by stage of disease this benefit was seen primarily after resection of stage IIIA cancers [1].

The ALPI trial was published in 2003 and studied the effect of adjuvant mitomycin, vindesine, and cisplatin after resection of NSCLC. Total accrual was 1209 patients, 39% had stage I disease, ratio of IA and IB patients unknown. Overall, ALPI failed to show any survival advantage for adjuvant mitomycin, vindesine, and cisplatin in the populations studied. For stages I (A and B) on this trial, the addition of mitomycin, vindesine, and cisplatin chemotherapy gave a hazard ratio for death at 97, with a 95% confidence interval ranging from 0.71 to 1.33 [5].

At the American Society of Clinical Oncology (ASCO) meeting in 2006, the Lung Adjuvant Cisplatin Evaluation (LACE) presented a pooled analysis of the individual patient data from the IALT, ALPI, ANITA, National Cancer Institute of Canada (NCIC) Br10, and Big Lung Trial studies. This analysis reviewed the data of 4584 patients who had been randomized to receive or not receive some form of adjuvant cisplatin-based chemotherapy after surgery. With a median follow-up of just over 5 years, LACE calculated that adjuvant cisplatin-based chemotherapy after resection of stage IA NSCLC was of no benefit, with a hazard ration for death at 1.41 and a 95% confidence interval ranging from 0.96 to 2.09 [4].

Stage IB

Stage IB disease was included in the populations studied in the IALT, NCIC Br 10, and ANITA trials [1–3] and made up the exclusive population studied in the Cancer and Leukemia Group B (CALGB) 9336 study (see Table 1) [6].

In IALT, about 25% of patients had stage IB disease. The hazard ratio (HR) of death was 0.95

E-mail address: eric.vallieres@swedish.org

Table 1
A summary of the recent European and North American trials that have studied the role adjuvant chemotherapy after the complete resection of stage I non–small cell lung carcinoma

Study	Overall results HR (CI)	Stage IA (N)	Stage IA results HR (CI)	Stage IB (N)	Stage IB results HR (CI)
IALT	0.86, $P < .03$	183	NA	498	0.95 (0.74–1.23)
NCIC, Br10	0.69, $P = .04$	Not tested	—	219	0.94 (NA)
ANITA	0.79, $P = .013$	Not tested	—	301	1.10 (0.76–1.57)
CALGB 9633	0.80, $P = .10$	Not tested	—	384	0.80 (0.6–1.07)
LACE	0.89, $P = .004$		1.41 (0.96–2.09)		0.93 (0.78–1.10)

with the use of a cisplatin doublet after surgery in these patients, with a 95% confidence interval ranging from 0.74 to 1.23 [1].

The results of NCIC Br 10 trial were first reported at ASCO 2004 and then published in 2005 [2]. A total of 482 patients were randomized to receive four cycles of adjuvant cisplatin and vinorelbine chemotherapy or not after complete resection of stages IB and II NSCLC. It took 7 years to complete this trial that showed an absolute overall survival advantage of 15% ($P = .03$) with the use of adjuvant cisplatin and vinorelbine after surgery. Nearly half of the patients in Br 10 (45%) had stage IB disease. Subgroup analysis by stage, however, suggested no benefit for adjuvant chemotherapy in stage IB disease with a hazard ratio for death just barely under 1 at 0.96 (Fig. 1).

One year later, the ANITA trial was reported at ASCO 2005. This study randomized 840 patients with stage IB, II, or IIIA disease to receive or not receive adjuvant cisplatin and vinorelbine after complete resection. Once again, the patients who received adjuvant systemic therapy came out on top with an 8.6% higher 5-year survival. A separate analysis, however, limited to the 301 (36%) patients with stage IB disease failed to show a benefit for adjuvant chemotherapy in this subset of the population studied [3].

The only completed trial to date that has studied the role of adjuvant chemotherapy exclusively in resected IB disease is the CALGB 9633 trial. After 7 years of accrual, a total of 384 patients with completely resected pT2N0 NSCLC were randomized to receive or not receive four cycles of adjuvant carboplatin and paclitaxel chemotherapy. When the preliminary results of this trial were reported in 2004, there was statistically significant evidence that adjuvant carboplatin and paclitaxel chemotherapy improved the 4-year survival by 12% ($P = .028$) [6]. Updated results reported at ASCO 2006,

however, showed a trend toward improvement in overall survival that had lost its statistical significance (HR = 0.80; 90% confidence interval 0.6–1.07; $P = .10$) with 5-year survivals of 60% and 57% in the respective arms ($P = .32$) [7]. A subset analysis of CALGB 9633 is said to suggest that a significant and positive effect of adjuvant chemotherapy is preserved, however, in tumors larger than 4 cm in size.

The LACE pooled analysis also addresses stage IB patients. Unfortunately, LACE showed a hazard ratio for death of 0.93 with a 95% confidence interval of 0.78 to 1.10, failing to show a significant survival benefit with adjuvant cisplatin chemotherapy in resected IB disease [4].

To date, on trial, the use of adjuvant chemotherapy has failed to show a survival benefit after the complete resection of stage IB disease: subset analysis of the three positive trials supporting the use of adjuvant cisplatin chemotherapy (IALT, NCIC Br10, and ANITA) have failed to see a benefit with IB disease, and the sole trial that exclusively targeted these patients seems to have lost its early promising significance (CALGB 9366). It is possible that adjuvant chemotherapy could be beneficial for patients with resected stage IB disease just as it has been shown to be in stages II and IIIA disease, but that the numbers of IB patients in the completed studies have been so far too small, and as such these trials were underpowered to address this question. The largest number of IB patients in any of these trials was only 498 (see Table 1).

Japan and adjuvant tegafur and uracil

For many years, Japanese investigators have studied the role of the combination of tegafur and uracil (1:4 ratio) (UFT) in the adjuvant setting after resection of early stage NSCLC. UFT is an

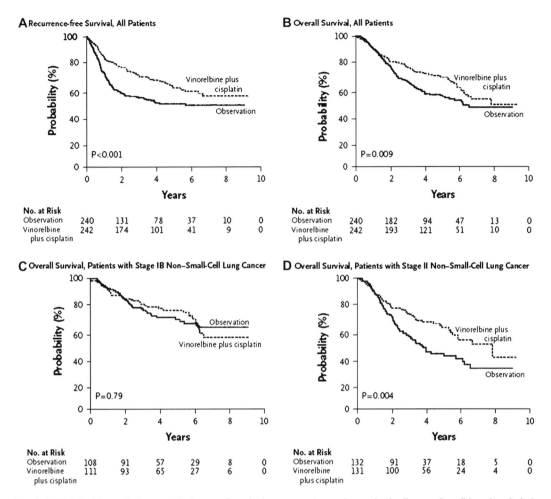

Fig. 1. NCIC Br 10, survival curves. Estimates of survival among patients who received adjuvant vinorelbine plus cisplatin and those who underwent observation alone. Note on panel C the lack of survival advantage seen with adjuvant chemotherapy after resection of IB NSCLC. (*From* Winton TL, Livingston R, Johnson D, et al. Vinorelbine plus cisplatin versus observation in resected NSCLC. N Engl J Med 2005;352:2595; with permission. Copyright © 2005, Massachusetts Medical Society.)

oral agent: tegafur gets converted into 5-fluorouracil, whereas uracil inhibits the enzymes that metabolize 5-fluorouracil, leading to enhanced antitumor activity. This 5-fluorouracil analogue has not been approved in the United States despite widespread approval elsewhere.

The West Japan Study Group for Lung Cancer Surgery reported in 1996 a three-arm trial where 310 patients with completely resected stages I to III NSCLC were randomized to observation only, adjuvant cisplatin-vindesine followed by oral UFT for 1 year, or UFT alone for 1 year. The two UFT arms did significantly better than the observation arm [8]. Subsequent subset analysis of this trial showed no statistically significant difference in the overall survival of patients with

squamous cell carcinoma between the two groups ($P = .24$). In contrast, patients with adenocarcinoma in the UFT group had a significantly better survival than those in the control group ($P = .009$). In addition, most patients with adenocarcinoma had stage I disease [9].

These observations led to another trial first reported at ASCO 2003 and published in 2004 [10]. This 979-patient trial by the Japan Lung Cancer Research Group targeted patients with completely resected stage I adenocarcinoma to receive or not receive oral UFT for 2 years. Most patients had T1N0 disease (N = 717 [73%]), and of these 412 were 2 cm or less in size. With a median follow-up of 6 years, there was a statistically significant improvement in survival in the UFT arm with a hazard ratio of death falling at 0.71 (0.52–0.98; $P = .04$). This effect was most pronounced for T2N0 tumors where the hazard ratio of death fell to 0.48 (0.21–0.81; $P = .005$) (Fig. 2). This benefit was not observed with stage IA lesions, which were predominantly of 2 cm or less in size on this study, but survival trends were noted for T1 lesions greater than or equal to 2 cm in size.

Finally, a meta-analysis of six adjuvant UFT trials in early disease was reported at ASCO 2004 and published in 2005. This included 2003 patients; most had stage I disease (96%) and were adenocarcinoma (85%). At 7 years, overall survival rates were 69.5% and 76.5% in the surgery-alone group and in the surgery plus UFT group, respectively, showing a significant survival benefit in the surgery plus UFT group. The overall pooled hazard ratio was 0.74, and its 95% confidence interval was 0.61 to 0.88 ($P = .001$). The number of squamous cell cancer in this analysis was too small to allow any conclusions, but this meta-analysis concluded that long-term treatment with UFT for 1 to 2 years was effective as postoperative adjuvant therapy in a Japanese patient population composed primarily of stage I adenocarcinoma patients [11]. At the ASCO 2004 presentation, Hamada and coworkers [12] also presented an exploratory analysis of the effect of adjuvant UFT in T1 tumors by size. He noted a statistically significant improvement in the 7-year survival with the use of adjuvant UFT for tumors of 2 to 3 cm (N = 599; $P = .0157$), an effect not seen with tumors less than 2 cm in size (N = 670; $P = .357$).

The future of adjuvant chemotherapy trials in stage I disease

The 5-year survival rates of resected stage IA and IB diseases are around 67% and 57%, respectively [13], translating into the fact that only about a third of patients with stage IA are at risk, close to 50% with stage IB. Stratification of patients' prognosis using solely the TNM staging system does not allow one to differentiate between the patients with stage I who are and who are not at risk. Despite the relatively small number of patients with stage I disease included in the competed trials to date, it is very possible that a positive effect for adjuvant chemotherapy in the treatment of resected stage I patients would have been seen if inclusion in these trials could have been restricted to patients at higher risk.

There is a growing literature supporting the use of genomics and proteomics to characterize lung cancers and their prognosis further (Fig. 3A) [14–16]. Still considered experimental, the application of these technologies is likely to become widespread in the near future. The next generation of trials exploring the potential benefit of adjuvant chemotherapy in early stage NSCLC will likely

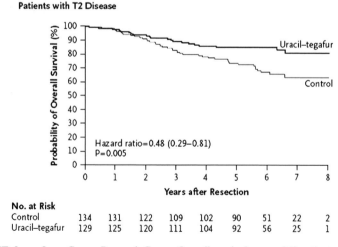

Patients with T2 Disease

No. at Risk

Control	134	131	122	109	102	90	51	22	2
Uracil–tegafur	129	125	120	111	104	92	56	25	1

Fig. 2. Adjuvant UFT: Japan Lung Cancer Research Group. Overall survival among 263 patients with T2N0 completely resected adenocarcinoma disease who were randomly assigned to the uracil-tegafur group and the control group. The hazard ratios indicate the risk of death in the uracil-tegafur group as compared with the control group. (*From* Kato H, Ichinose Y, Ohta M, et al. A randomized trial of adjuvant chemotherapy with uracil-tegafur for adenocarcinoma of the lung. N Engl J Med 2004;350:1717; with permission. Copyright © 2004, Massachusetts Medical Society.)

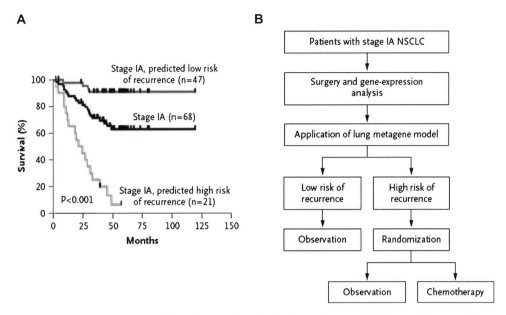

Fig. 3. (*A*) Genomics to predict prognosis. Kaplan-Meier survival estimates for a combined group of patients with stage IA disease from three unrelated cohorts (Duke, ACOSOG, CALGB) and the subgroups predicted to have either a high probability (>0.5) or a low probability (≤ 0.5) of recurrence as per the application of the lung metagene model. (*B*) Proposal for future adjuvant chemotherapy trial guided by genomics prognostication. This illustrates a possible design of a planned prospective, phase III clinical trial involving patients with stage IA NSCLC to evaluate the performance of the metagene model. (*From* Potti A, Mukherjee S, Petersen R, et al. A genomic strategy to refine prognosis in early-stage non–small-cell lung cancer. N Engl J Med 2006;355:578; with permission. Copyright © 2006, Massachusetts Medical Society.)

incorporate some genomics or proteomics to refine the groups at risk and possibly determine who should and should not be considered for adjuvant chemotherapy (Fig. 3B) [14]. Such a strategy could permit statistically significant trials to be of relatively small size and allow them to be completed in a more rapid time than in the past.

Pharmacogenomics is another science that may become an integral part of the future adjuvant therapy trials in early stage NSCLC (Fig. 4) [17]. For example, set tumor markers could help determine sensitivity to particular chemotherapy agents and the presence or absence of these markers could help determine which drugs to use or to avoid in patients.

Summary

Based on the limited data presented, in North America and in Europe, one cannot recommend the routine use of adjuvant systemic chemotherapy after the complete resection of stages IA and IB NSCLC. It is possible that the completed trials have been underpowered to see a survival

advantage in this patient population that carries a better prognosis overall. The data from Japan are certainly intriguing and bring a potentially new adjuvant strategy for these patients: low-dose, long-term, well-tolerated adjuvant oral therapy. Adjuvant UFT needs to be studied outside of Japan before this strategy gets adopted worldwide. In 2007, in Japan, adjuvant UFT is often recommended after the complete resection of stages IA and IB adenocarcinoma.

One also realizes that not every resected stage I tumor carries the same prognosis, a fact that most trials have not taken into consideration. Despite the lack of trial results to support adjuvant chemotherapy in stage IA and IB diseases, however, outside of a clinical trial setting, it is probably reasonable to consider the possibility of adjuvant systemic chemotherapy in the individualized healthy younger patient whose resected tumor exhibited poor prognostic histologic findings, such as lymphovascular invasion, larger size, or even high fluorodeoxyglucose avidity on preoperative positron emission tomography scan [18]. Ideally, however, these patients should all be considered to participate in the next generation

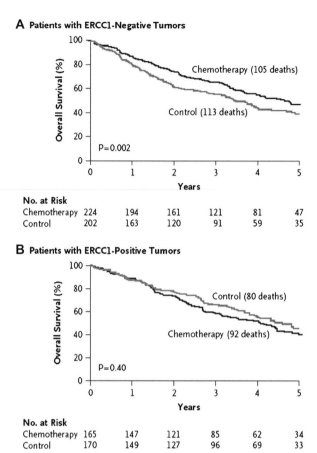

Fig. 4. Proteomics predicting the response to cisplatin-based chemotherapy given in the adjuvant setting in the IALT study. (*A*) Overall survival according to treatment in patients with ERCC1-negative tumors. The adjusted hazard ratio for death in the chemotherapy group, as compared with the control group, was 0.65 (95% CI, 0.50–0.86; P = .002). (*B*) Overall survival according to treatment in patients with ERCC1-positive tumors. The adjusted hazard ratio for death in the chemotherapy group, as compared with the control group, was 1.14 (95% CI, 0.84–1.55; P = .40). (*From* Olaussen KA, Dunant A, Fouret P, et al. DNA repair by ERCC1 in non–small-cell lung cancer and cisplatin-based adjuvant chemotherapy. N Engl J Med 2006;355:989; with permission. Copyright © 2006, Massachusetts Medical Society.)

of trials exploring the strategy of adjuvant therapy in the management of completely resected stage I NSCLC.

Reference

[1] The International Adjuvant Lung Cancer Trial Collaborative Group. Cisplatin-based adjuvant chemotherapy in patients with completely resected NSCLC. N Engl J Med 2004;350:351–60.

[2] Winton TL, Livingston R, Johnson D, et al. Vinorelbine plus cisplatin vs. observation in resected NSCLC. N Engl J Med 2005;352:2589–97.

[3] Douillard J, Rosell R, Delena M, et al. Adjuvant vinorelbine plus cisplatin versus observation in patients with completely resected stage IB-IIIA non-small-cell lung cancer (Adjuvant Navelbine International Trialist Association [ANITA]): a randomised controlled trial. Lancet Oncol 2006;7(9):719–27.

[4] Pignon JP, Tribodet H, Scagliotti GV, et al. On behalf of the LACE Collaborative Group. Lung Adjuvant Cisplatin Evaluation (LACE): a pooled analysis of five randomized clinical trials including 4,584 patients. ASCO Annual Meeting Proceedings. J Clin Oncol 2006;24:7008.

[5] Scagliotti GV, Fossati R, Torri V, et al. For the Adjuvant Lung project Italy/EORTC. Randomized study of adjuvant chemotherapy for completely resected stage I, II or IIIA NSCLC. J Nat Cancer Inst 2003;95:1453–61.

[6] Strauss GM, Herndon J, Maddaus MA, et al. Randomized clinical trial of adjuvant chemotherapy

with paclitaxel and carboplatin following resection in stage IB non-small cell lung cancer (NSCLC): report of Cancer and Leukemia Group B (CALGB) Protocol 9633. ASCO Annual Meeting Proceedings. J Clin Oncol 2004;22:7019.

[7] Strauss GM, Herndon J, Maddaus MA, et al. Adjuvant chemotherapy in stage IB NSCLC: update of CALGB protocol 9633. ASCO Annual Meeting Proceedings. J Clin Oncol 2006;24:7007.

[8] Wada H, Hitomi S, Teramatsu T, et al. Adjuvant chemotherapy after complete resection in non-small cell lung cancer. J Clin Oncol 1996;14:1048–52.

[9] Okimoto N, Soejima R, Teramatsu T, et al. A randomized controlled postoperative adjuvant chemotherapy trial of CDDP + VDS + UFT and UFT alone in comparison with operation only for non-small cell lung carcinomas (second study). Japanese Journal of Lung Cancer 1996;36:863–78.

[10] Kato H, Ichinose Y, Ohta M, et al. A randomized trial of adjuvant chemotherapy with uracil–tegafur for adenocarcinoma of the lung. N Engl J Med 2004;350:1713–21.

[11] Hamada C, Tanaka F, Ohta M, et al. Meta-analysis of postoperative adjuvant chemotherapy with tegafur-uracil in non–small-cell lung cancer. J Clin Oncol 2005;23:4999–5006.

[12] Hamada C, Ohta M, Wada S, et al. Survival benefit of oral UFT for adjuvant chemotherapy after completely resected NSCLC. ASCO Annual Meeting Proceedings. J Clin Oncol 2004;22:7002.

[13] Mountain CF. Revisions in the international system for staging lung cancer. Chest 1997;111:1710–7.

[14] Potti A, Mukherjee S, Petersen R, et al. A genomic strategy to refine prognosis in early-stage non–small-cell lung cancer. N Engl J Med 2006;355:570–80.

[15] Chen HY, Yu SL, Chen CH, et al. A five-gene signature and clinical outcome in non–small-cell lung cancer. N Engl J Med 2007;356:11–20.

[16] Zheng Z, Chen T, Li X, et al. DNA synthesis and repair genes RRM1 and ERCC1 in lung cancer. N Engl J Med 2007;356:800–8.

[17] Olaussen KA, Dunant A, Fouret P, et al. DNA repair by erccl in non–small-cell lung cancer and cisplatin-based adjuvant chemotherapy. N Engl J Med 2006;355:983–91.

[18] Cerfolio RJ, Bryant AS, Ohja B, et al. The maximum standardized uptake values on positron emission tomography of a non–small cell lung cancer predict stage, recurrence, and survival. J Thorac Cardiovasc Surg 2005;130:151–9.

ELSEVIER
SAUNDERS

Thorac Surg Clin 17 (2007) 287–299

THORACIC
SURGERY
CLINICS

Adjuvant Chemotherapy and the Role of Chemotherapy Resistance Testing for Stage I Non–Small Cell Lung Cancer

Thomas A. d'Amato, MD, PhD

*Section of Thoracic Surgery, Jefferson Medical College of Thomas Jefferson University,
1025 Walnut Street, Suite 607, Philadelphia, PA 19107, USA*

Lung cancer claimed nearly 162,460 lives in 2006, accounting for more cancer-related deaths than breast and prostate cancers combined [1]. For early stage non–small cell lung cancer (NSCLC), surgical resection remains the standard, yet the expected 5-year survival ranges only from 25% to 65% in patients with completely resected disease [2]. Administration of adjuvant chemotherapy accounts for a small but significant (4%–15%) improvement in survival [3–6], supporting its use in patients with stage II and IIIA disease. With the exclusion of patients with stage IA NSCLC, an added benefit for resected stage 1B patients remains unproved [7].

Empiric use of postoperative cytotoxic agents, particularly for early stage disease, is a "shotgun" approach taken with no prior knowledge of a patient's tumor-specific biology to predict its clinical efficacy or necessity. Tumor resistance to chemotherapy results in few patients who can be cured with adjuvant chemotherapy. Because all antineoplastic agents have significant adverse effects, then most patients given adjuvant chemotherapy endure toxicity without a survival benefit. Distinguishing between patients with a high risk for early recurrence and those patients with a long disease-free interval following resection alone, and identifying those who may respond to adjuvant therapy, are topics of great interest and intense

study in this new era of pharmacogenomics. Genetic and phenotypic analysis, prognostic molecular marker testing, and chemotherapy resistance assays all share a cognate role in the development of individualized patient care algorithms.

This article describes the current clinical application of in vitro chemotherapy resistance testing of patient tumors. The staggering prevalence of NSCLC in vitro tumor resistance is reviewed, and the potential role of the extreme drug resistant (EDR) assay in both clinical and laboratory investigations are discussed.

Chemotherapy for stage 1 lung cancer and application of the extreme drug resistant assay

Recommendations for platinum-based adjuvant chemotherapy after complete resection of stage IB to IIIA NSCLC have increased following recent reports of four randomized clinical trials (Table 1) [3–7]. All of these adjuvant trials included stage 1 patients; however, none revealed a significant improvement in patients with stage 1 disease. Despite adjuvant cytotoxic therapy, at least 85% of patients did not benefit. All chemotherapy regimens, however, were associated with predictable toxicity in 23% to 86% of patients [3–6]. Since 2004, the controversy regarding the universal application of adjuvant chemotherapy following resection of stage 1B disease continued after a 12% improvement in overall survival at 4 years was observed in the CALGB 9633 trial among patients receiving adjuvant carboplatin and paclitaxel [4]. Subsequent subset analysis of

---

The author discloses a consultant relationship with Oncotech, Inc., Tustin, CA.

E-mail address: thomas.damato@jefferson.edu

Table 1
Adjuvant chemotherapy trials for non–small cell lung cancer: stage response and toxicity

Adjuvant trial	Regimen planned	Stage included	Stage response	Patients completing therapy (%)	Grade 3 or 4 toxicity (%)	Chemotherapy-related deaths
IALT	Cisplatin + VP-16 or Vinca alkaloid	I, II, III	IIIA	628/851 (74)	23[a]	7
CALBG 9633	Carboplatin + paclitaxel	IB	NS[c]	68/124 (55)	36[b]	0
JBR-10	Cisplatin + vinorelbine	IB, II	II	110/242 (48)[d,e]	73	2
ANITA[f]	Cisplatin + vinorelbine	IB, II, IIIA	II, IIIA	368/407 (90)[g]	86	5

[a] Only grade 4 toxicity reported.

[b] Toxicity data available for 149 (86%) of 173 patients randomized, but data were available in only 124 (72%) of 173 patients who received chemotherapy and only 55% received full dose.

[c] NS: Stage response was underpowered to achieve significance.

[d] Dose reduction was required for 77%.

[e] 65% completed three cycles.

[f] Percent of patients receiving chemotherapy following randomization: only 56% completed vinorelbine therapy, 76% completed cisplatin therapy.

[g] 39% received chemotherapy at relapse.

these data revealed that only patients with a tumor size greater than 4.5 cm benefited from adjuvant chemotherapy and the CALGB 9633 trial was underpowered to achieve statistical significance [7]. Despite these updated data, adjuvant therapy is still often recommended for selected stage 1B believed to be at high risk for recurrence [7], but it remains not indicated for completely resected stage 1A disease [3].

Because of the increased frequency of recommendations to prescribe adjuvant chemotherapy in resected NSCLC, I developed an interest in chemotherapy resistance testing. Through collaborative efforts in a multidisciplinary clinic at Thomas Jefferson University Hospital, medical oncology colleagues are now more receptive to this existing technology. The purpose of using the EDR assay is to avoid unnecessary toxicity (particularly in early stage disease) by simply avoiding ineffective agents, and when feasible, to tailor chemotherapy regimens based on in vitro resistance testing of fresh tissue. It is hoped that other medical oncologists will be encouraged to consider resistance testing as part of their armamentarium to estimate clinical response to cytotoxic agents. Despite these efforts, some oncologists have continued skepticism, in part because of underappreciated technical developments and concepts that distinguish between chemosensitivity and chemoresistance.

Resistance versus sensitivity, the extreme drug resistant assay, and predicting clinical response

A recent review and technology assessment by the American Association of Clinical Oncology (ASCO) does not endorse the routine use of chemotherapy resistance and sensitivity assays [8,9]. Unfortunately, these authors failed to acknowledge several shortcomings of abandoned technology, and in their report did not distinguish salient differences between sensitivity and resistance testing, and failed to review much of the current literature supporting chemotherapy resistance testing [10,11].

Chemotherapy sensitivity and resistance assays performed with older clonogenic assays relied on brief exposures to chemotherapy at or below peak serum concentrations; frequently used cell culture techniques permitting growth of stromal elements; required long incubation times, limiting clinical usefulness; and often used inaccurate manual cell-counting methods, resulting in erroneous data. Over several decades, advances in cell culture technology, test availability, reliability, and reproducibility of measurable end points (cellular proliferation) have contributed to the accuracy of chemotherapy-resistant assays. This prompted the Medicare approval of in vitro chemotherapy resistance (not sensitivity) testing well before the ASCO technology assessment was published [12]. Basic principles regarding the predictive accuracy of measuring resistance compared with estimating sensitivity, and perhaps the oncology communities' desire to know "which agent will work," may have limited the widespread application of chemotherapy resistance testing with the exception of ovarian cancer.

Conceptually, a relatively simple in vitro biologic test that is a good example of a resistance assay is the Kirby-Bauer bacterial culture and sensitivity test. This assay has a predictive accuracy of 90% true-positives (clinical resistance to therapy) versus only 60% accuracy in predicting true-negatives (ie, clinical sensitivity). For example, if a bacterial culture grows in the presence of an antimicrobial, it is unlikely that a patient will respond to therapy, whereas "sensitive" bacteria in culture may not equate with clinical response to therapy up to 40% of the time. Ironically, it is named a bacterial sensitivity test, but clinicians actually rely on its ability accurately to detect resistance [13]. Modern chemotherapy resistance testing is quite similar in concept.

The most validated method to determine in vitro chemotherapy resistance in human tumors is the EDR Assay (Oncotech, Tustin, California).

Viable human tumors are dissociated into single cells and small cellular aggregates, which maintain cell-cell interaction. This is more apt to represent the patient's tumor than the clonogenic assay. Cultured cells are exposed to chemotherapeutic agents at concentrations 5 to 10 times the peak serum levels attained in patients and cellular proliferation is measured by ^{3}H-thymidine uptake [14]. Positive controls (supralethal cisplatin resulting in 100% cell death) and negative controls (media exposed only) are used to determine the percent colony inhibition (PCI) by an individual drug compared with media-exposed cultures correcting for positive controls (Fig. 1).

From a historical database of over 140,000 human tumors of varied histology submitted for the EDR assay, the PCI values are compared with the median PCI of the entire population for any given drug tested. Tumors exhibiting PCI values one standard deviation above the population median are defined as low drug resistant (LDR); tumors with PCI values between the population median and one standard deviation below the median are defined as intermediate drug resistant (IDR); and tumors with PCI values that are one

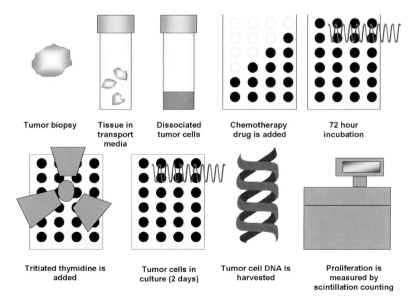

Fig. 1. Methodology of the EDR assay. Fresh tumor obtained as a surgical biopsy is suspended in tissue culture medium and transported overnight to the central laboratory. Specimens are disassociated into single cells and small cellular aggregates and cultured as described previously [12]. Tumor cultures are exposed to chemotherapeutic agents at final concentrations 5 to 10 times higher than expected in vivo peak plasma levels. Following a 72-hour exposure, 5 μCi of ^{3}H-thymidine (Amersham Biosciences, Piscataway, New Jersey) is added and incubation is continued for an additional 48 hours. Cell suspensions are harvested and cellular proliferation is determined by ^{3}H-thymidine incorporation into DNA and measured by scintillation counting (Beckman-Coulter, Fullerton, California). (*Courtesy of* Oncotech, Inc., Tustin, CA.)

standard deviation below the median PCI are defined as EDR.

The EDR assay was developed accurately to measure in vitro resistance without reference to either in vitro or clinical sensitivity. With chemosensitivity assays, an assumption is made that brief exposure to concentrations of chemotherapeutic drugs, at or below clinical peak plasma levels, models the tumors in vivo exposure. Such factors as interindividual metabolism, tumor vascular supply, and anatomic permeability barriers, however, affect tumor chemotherapy exposure (concentration × time). These potentially important individual patient biologic determinants of response to cytotoxic agents are virtually impossible to assimilate in the in vitro setting. Additionally, pharmacokinetic factors varying from patient to patient, such as absorption, activation, and elimination of a cytotoxic drug, can cause significant differences in tumor drug exposure, resulting in differences in clinical response even when tumors in an in vitro setting may be equally chemosensitive. These factors significantly limit the accuracy to predict "clinical sensitivity" to any cytotoxic agent [13]. In contrast, the EDR assay tumor exposure to antineoplastic agents is long (120 hours) at concentrations that approximate or exceed peak plasma levels. The tumor cell exposure is many times greater than levels achieved in the patient. If the percentage of a specific tumor's growth (measured by DNA proliferation) in the EDR assay is one standard deviation below the median inhibition determined for thousands of tumors, then that tumor is considered to be resistant to that drug [13,14].

The predictive accuracy (posttest probability) of the EDR assay is not only a function of tumor exposure, but also the expected response (pretest) probability of a given patient to a specific agent. This bayesian statistical model was used by Kern and Weisenthal [14] in their retrospective chart review of 450 patients correlating assay results with clinical response. Only 1 of the 127 patients with extreme drug resistance responded to chemotherapy. In NSCLC, only 2 of 20 patient's tumors exhibiting in vitro intermediate or extreme drug resistance responded. Subset analysis comparing tumor types expected to be sensitive and those expected to be resistant revealed that the EDR assay's ability to identify extreme drug resistance and to predict treatment failure (negative posttest probability of response) was independent of the expected (pretest) probability of response. The ability of the EDR assay to detect tumor

resistance to a particular chemotherapeutic agent was over 99% specific [13,14].

Chemotherapy resistance in non–small cell lung cancer

We recently reported the prevalence of in vitro extreme chemotherapy resistance in 3042 resected NSCLC tumors [15]. For chemotherapeutic agents used as first-line therapy in the most recent adjuvant chemotherapy clinical trials, extreme or intermediate drug resistance of human NSCLC tumor cultures exposed to carboplatin was found in 1056 (68%) of 1565; to cisplatin in 1409 (63%) of 2227; to etoposide in 1581 (63%) of 2505; to navelbine in 603 (42%) of 1444; to paclitaxel in 689 (40%) of 1706; to gemcitabine in 594 (72%) of 823; to taxotere in 273 (525) of 521; and to topotecan in 280 (31%) of 896 of NSCLC cultures tested (Fig. 2).

Subsequently, we analyzed over 4571 NSCLC specimens, and evaluated patient tumor cultures that were assayed separately against platin agents, cisplatin plus carboplatin, and vinca alkaloids, vinblastine plus vincristine to measure concordant resistant patterns for like agents [16]. Concordant resistance patterns were determined by plotting PCI values for individual tumors tested with the first drug (ordinate) versus the same tumor tested against the second drug (abscissa). Assuming that some frequency of EDR, IDR, and LDR to any given drug exists in a population of separate tumors tested against one drug, if a set of tumors is tested against two independent drugs, then a 3×3 matrix can be created where nine possible resistance patterns are possible for the population. Within this population, each tumor has a unique resistance to each agent; for example, one subset of tumors will be EDR to both drugs and a subset will be LDR to both drugs. Seven other combinations of EDR, IDR, and LDR are possible. From this matrix, subpopulations exhibiting any EDR plus IDR combination to both drugs tested and those exhibiting EDR or IDR to at least one agent were calculated. Correlation coefficients from scatterplot analysis using linear regression analysis were performed with the Spotfire statistical package (Spotfire, Sommerville, Massachusetts) to illustrate tumor resistance patterns for any given doublet pair analyzed.

For cisplatin and carboplatin, 1099 specimens were tested separately to both agents and showed similar distributions of drug resistance (R = 0.76).

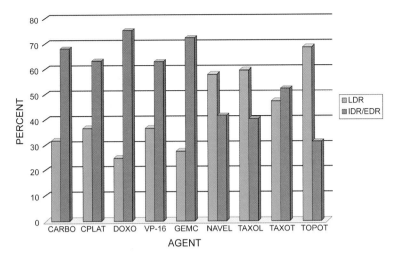

Fig. 2. Prevalence of in vitro chemotherapy resistance for resected NSCLC specimens. The percent of patient NSCLC tumor cultures (N = 3042) exhibiting EDR-IDR or LDR in the EDR assay are shown for chemotherapy agents: carboplatin (CARBO), N = 1565; cisplatin (CPLAT), N = 2227; doxorubicin (DOXO), N = 1471; etoposide (VP 16), N = 2505; gemcitabine (GMCB), N = 823; paclitaxel (TAXOL), N = 1706; taxotere (TAXOT), N = 521; and topotecan (TOPOT), N = 896. (*Adapted from* d'Amato TA, Landreneau RJ, McKenna RJ, et al. Prevalence of in vitro extreme chemotherapy resistance in resected non-small lung cancer. Ann Thorac Surg 2006;81:443; with permission.)

For the vinca alkaloids, 28 cultures were assayed with both agents and resistance profiles correlated (R = 0.92) (Fig. 3). Little correlation was noted for the paired combinations carboplatin plus paclitaxel and the drug combinations tested with cisplatin: navelbine, docetaxel, or gemcitabine. For 1523 tumors separately tested with carboplatin and paclitaxel (R = 0.189), 80 (5%) were EDR and 393 (26%) were LDR to both drugs. Combined IDR and EDR tumors were observed in 422 (28%) of the population and 1130 (74%) were IDR or EDR to at least one agent (Fig. 4A). In 1314 cultures tested for cisplatin and navelbine (R = 0.018), 32 (2%) were EDR

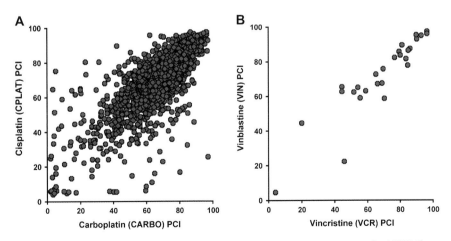

Fig. 3. Correlation and concurrent chemotherapy resistance illustrating congruent patterns for NSCLC tumor cultures exposed in separate assays to like agents. (*A*) Cisplatin and carboplatin (N = 1099; R = 0.76) and (*B*) vinblastine and vincristine (N = 28; R = 0.92) are shown as PCI for each drug tested. Each data point (jittered for clarity) represents the combined in vitro response for a single tumor culture. (*Adapted from* d'Amato TA, Landreneau RJ, Ricketts W. Chemotherapy resistance and oncogene expression in non-small cell lung cancer. J Thorac Cardiovasc Surg 2007;133:355; with permission.)

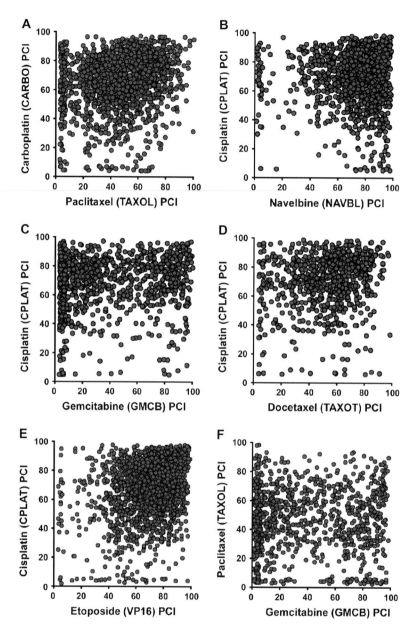

Fig. 4. Concurrent chemotherapy resistance patterns for NSCLC tumor cultures exposed in separate assays to one of four standard platinum-based chemotherapy doublets. (*A*) Carboplatin and paclitaxel (N = 1523; R = 0.189); (*B*) cisplatin and navelbine (N = 1314; R = 0.018); (*C*) cisplatin and gemcitabine (N = 944; R = 0.09); (*D*) cisplatin and docetaxel (N = 741; R = 0.182); (*E*) cisplatin and etoposide (N = 2018; R = 0.279); and (*F*) gemcitabine and paclitaxel (N = 693; R = 0.04) are shown for each pair as PCI for each drug tested. Each data point (jittered for clarity) represents the combined in vitro response for a single tumor culture. (*Adapted from* d'Amato TA, Landreneau RJ, Ricketts W, et al. Chemotherapy resistance and oncogene expression in non-small cell lung cancer. J Thorac Cardiovasc Surg 2007; 133:355; with permission.)

and 418 (32%) were LDR to both. Combined IDR and EDR tumor cultures comprised 263 (20%) of the population and 896 (68%) were IDR or EDR to at least one drug (Fig. 4B). For

cisplatin and gemcitabine, of 994 cultures tested (R = 0.09), 136 (14%) were EDR and 110 (11%) were LDR to both. Combined IDR and EDR tumor cultures comprised 439 (44%) of the population and 884 (89%) were resistant to at least one (Fig. 4C). For cisplatin and docetaxel, of 741 cultures tested (R = 0.182), 35 (5%) were EDR and (32%) were LDR to both. Combined IDR and EDR tumor cultures comprised 202 (27%) of the population and 507 (68%) were resistant to at least one (Fig. 4D). For cisplatin and etoposide, of 2018 tumor cultures tested (R = 0.279), 95 (5%) were EDR and 426 (21%) were LDR to both agents. Combined IDR and EDR cultures comprised 478 (24%) of the population and 1572 (79%) were resistant to at least one (Fig. 4E). For the nonplatin doublet, gemcitabine and paclitaxel, of 693 cultures tested (R = 0.04), 47 (7%) were EDR and 294 (25%) were LDR to both. Combined IDR and EDR tumor cultures comprised 439 (37%) of the population and 579 (84%) were resistant to at least one (Fig. 4F).

Notwithstanding the potential for synergy among paired agents, had these agents been tested together, these in vitro data suggest that many patients may benefit from only one of the two agents in doublet therapy and that simultaneous resistance occurs frequently, which may have profound clinical relevance. Mehta and coworkers [17] examined this phenomenon in breast cancer and found that the median time to disease progression and survival was significantly shorter for patients treated with any combination of agents exhibiting either extreme or intermediate in vitro drug resistance in comparison with patients having tumors with low in vitro resistance to both drugs. In vitro drug resistance correlated with a shorter survival similar to that associated with advanced stage or positive lymph node status. It is interesting to note that in our study, tumor resistance observed in doublet analysis is in parallel with the observed clinical response reported in the JBR.10 and ANITA trials, where the greatest survival advantage is reported with the cisplatin plus vinorelbine doublet [5,6,15,16].

Chemotherapy resistance in other solid tumors

In ovarian cancer, Holloway and coworkers [18] demonstrated that ovarian cancer patients' tumors exhibiting in vitro platinum resistance in the EDR assay had a significantly shortened progression-free and overall survival when treated with a platinum-based agent. Loizzi and colleagues [19] showed that patients with platinum-sensitive tumors treated with assay-directed therapy compared with patients treated with

empiric therapy had both a highly significant improvement in overall survival (assay directed, 90%; empiric therapy, 70%; P = .005) and 1-year progression-free survival (assay directed, 68%; empiric treatment, 16%; P = .0002).

Patients with recurrent malignant glioma were prospectively evaluated for irinotecan resistance [20] in a blinded study to predict the reliability of the EDR assay. Median time to progression for IDR-LDR cases was 3 months versus 6 weeks for EDR cases (P = .0288; hazards ratio = 3.06). A 13-week median survival for EDR cases was significantly shorter compared with 38 weeks for IDR-LDR cases (P = .029). The 100-day survival favored the IDR-LDR cases (P = .008).

The clinical observations of tumor unresponsiveness to chemotherapy correlating with in vitro resistance in ovarian, breast, and brain tissues supports the potential application of the EDR assay in NSCLC.

Clinical and scientific use of chemotherapy resistance testing

Because the prevalence of in vitro chemoresistance in resected NSCLC tumors is significant, unresponsiveness to a given platinum agent in patients with resistant tumors is likely. Therapeutic trends exist wherein a patient's tumor may be resistant to platinum in vitro, yet a platinum-based drug is given. Although this is consistent with current treatment algorithms, few patients benefit. We recommend that if a patient's tumor is less resistant to one platinum drug over another, then the least resistant platinum agent should be used.

In platinum-based doublet therapy, choosing the second agent by using resistance testing can help avoid one cytotoxic drug based on its in vitro ineffectiveness, and potentially select a more effective therapeutic option. For example, if a patient's tumor is extremely resistant to paclitaxel, navelbine may be substituted. Both alternatives are accepted second agents with expected similar survival statistics.

Finally, patients with metastatic disease or those undergoing salvage therapy may benefit most from deselecting one empiric chemotherapeutic drug when alternatives exist, thereby avoiding toxicity from ineffective second- or third-line therapies. In stage IV lung cancer patients, Schiller and coworkers [21] reported that none of four accepted empiric chemotherapy platinum doublets offered a significant survival advantage over another (Fig. 5), and the carboplatin plus paclitaxel doublet was chosen as the Eastern Cooperative Oncology Group standard because of its reduced toxicity. To avoid further unnecessary toxicity, stage IV NSCLC patients should have EDR testing to help choose the least resistant doublet in platinum-based therapy, to choose the best single agent, or to prescribe a nonplatinum drug combination.

Discovering tumor resistance: cell cultures, DNA, RNA, or protein?

The EDR assay, although specific for identifying tumor resistance, is limited by the need for fresh tissue. Some molecular diagnostic tests performed on archived specimens can be used to detect genetic abnormalities that impart resistance to cytotoxic drugs. For example, the abnormal expression of the ERCC1 gene was recently shown to correlate with platinum resistance. This discovery and the development and application of quantifying ERRC1 in NSCLC are noteworthy.

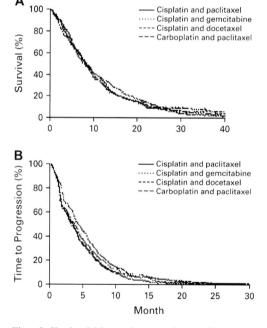

Fig. 5. Kaplan-Meier estimates of overall survival (*A*) and the time to progression of disease (*B*) in the ECOG study patients enrolled according to their assigned treatment. (*From* Schiller J, Harrington D, Belani C, et al. Comparison of four chemotherapy regimens for advanced non-small-cell lung cancer. N Engl J Med 2002; 346:92–8; with permission.)

RNA microdissected from archived tissue cell blocks was used to identify overexpression of ERCC1 in patient tumors where clinical unresponsiveness to cisplatin was observed [22]. This provided a proof of concept; however, its clinical applicability as a laboratory test is limited. RNA quality extracted from paraffin-embedded tissues is variable depending on the amount of RNAse degradation, which reduces the yield and integrity of the extracted RNA. The complexity of RNA analysis and its unavailability in most clinical laboratories currently limits its usefulness as a routine diagnostic test. The ability to identify abnormal overexpression of ERCC1, however, afforded the opportunity to develop a validated immunohistochemical assay based on antibodies to the ERCC1 protein. This technology was subsequently used reliably to detect abnormal expression of ERCC1 in archived tissues from paraffin blocks. NSCLC tumors from patients enrolled in the IALT trial were analyzed for ERCC1 by immunohistochemical methods. Those patients with high expression of ERCC1 who were treated with platinum had shorter survival times compared with patients in the chemotherapy arm having low ERCC1 expression [23]. This is an example where identification of abnormal ERCC1 gene expression by one method (using RNA technology) can be translated into a standardized inexpensive diagnostic test (immunohistochemical assay) that is used routinely by many clinical laboratories.

Gene expression profiles, based on RNA arrays that may refine estimates of prognosis in patients with resected NSCLC, have recently been identified [24,25] and include genes believed to impart tumor metastatic potential [25,26]. This technology, however, is not generally available as a diagnostic tool. Furthermore, the clinical reliability of an RNA array assay and its ability to predict prognosis or drug response to chemotherapy have recently been questioned, and may be inferior to usually applied clinical and pathologic features like gender and tumor histopathology [27].

Chemotherapy resistance testing creates a unique opportunity to use resistant tumors as surrogates to help identify specific genes that impart resistance to chemotherapeutics. This may streamline efforts to identify specific resistance gene expression profiles with RNA array analysis, or DNA array methods to identify specific gene amplifications, deletions, or rearrangements. Subsequently, specific diagnostic tests can be developed to predict accurately a patient's response to cytotoxic or targeted therapy.

We have recently used the EDR assay as a surrogate to identify NSCLC tumors resistant to paclitaxel. DNA was purified from tumors that exhibited EDR to paclitaxel and were analyzed by competitive genomic hybridization to DNA bacterial clones representing the entire human genome (Spectral Genomics, Houston, Texas). A molecular karyotype identified an amplification of sequences on chromosome 1q that was not only consistent among other paclitaxel-resistant NSCLC tumors but to breast and ovarian tumors exhibiting in vitro resistance to paclitaxel [28]. Subsequently, a specific DNA gene probe representing the chromosome 1q25 (Abbott Molecular, Deplanes, Illinois) was used to develop and validate a florescent in situ hybridization assay to screen patient tumors for paclitaxel resistance (Fig. 6). Using this technology, the association of 1q25 amplification, paclitaxel resistance, and clinical responsiveness can now be studied.

Competitive genomic hybridization arrays, RNA microarrays, and known clinical and histopathologic features should all be integrated into modern clinical trials designed to evaluate prognosis and response to therapy in NSCLC. The EDR assays ability reliably to detect in vitro resistance and its potential use as a surrogate for discovering genetic features that convey unresponsiveness to chemotherapy support its use in future cooperative group studies.

Planned and proposed clinical trials to estimate prognosis and response to adjuvant chemotherapy

Although fresh tissue specimens are generally available for chemotherapy resistance testing at the time of surgery, its application for the purpose of assay-directed treatment is currently lacking clinical validation in NSCLC, and may be yet another obstacle toward use of the EDR assay in clinical practice. The recent ASCO Technology Assessment [8] has recommended that future studies be designed comparing empiric chemotherapy with resistance assay–directed chemotherapy. Unfortunately, the general medical oncology community has yet to integrate this concept into any cooperative group trial [11]. Moreover, in a rebuttal to the ASCO report, Weiand [29], suggested that the clinical use of resistance testing be validated in a single-arm, noninterventional assay accuracy trial using two or more therapies known to have similar response rates to determine whether the assay is predictive of response. We agree with Weiand's assessment of this concept and encourage thoracic surgeons with access to fresh tumors to seize the opportunity to evaluate

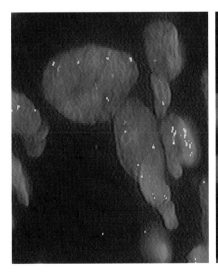 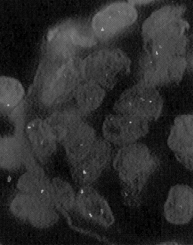

Fig. 6. Photomicrograph illustrating the florescent in situ hybridization (FISH) results for a non–small cell tumor exhibiting in vitro paclitaxel resistance in the EDR assay (original magnification ×400). A FISH probe representing human chromosome 1q25 (Abbott Molecular, Des Plaines, Illinois) exhibits green fluorescence and demonstrates gene amplification. Red florescence represents unamplified sequences on chromosome 1p36 and serves as an internal control. (*Courtesy of* Oncotech, Inc., Tustin, California.)

the predictive power of in vitro chemoresistance testing with the EDR assay by integrating it to both observational and randomized prospective trials.

Recently, clinicians at Duke University developed a lung metagene model, based on RNA microarray analysis, to predict which patients following complete resection for stage IA NSCLC are at risk for early recurrence [24,25]. This concept is discussed elsewhere in this issue. The results of this study have prompted the development of a CALGB randomized phase 3 clinical trial designed to evaluate the benefit of identifying a group of stage 1A NSCLC patients estimated to be at high risk for recurrence. Patients at high risk would be randomized to observation (the current standard for completely resected stage 1A disease), or to receive adjuvant platinum-based chemotherapy. Although this model may be an appropriate application of a genomic strategy to

estimate prognosis, by identifying early stage lung cancer patients who may benefit from adjuvant chemotherapy, it still involves empiric application of cytotoxic therapy. Nevertheless, it could potentially serve as a suitable platform to evaluate in vitro tumor resistance assays and to identify genes and tumor phenotypes associated with clinical resistance to chemotherapy. Certainly, this and other opportunities exist to validate chemotherapy resistance testing.

A phase 2 validation registry trial designed to measure outcome following empiric adjuvant chemotherapy in patients where the EDR assay is performed will evaluate standard of care platinum-based chemotherapy treatment in patients with tumors that exhibit platinum resistance. As a registry or validation trial, correlating the in vitro assay results to clinical responsiveness can be done either as a correlative study in a surgical trial, as a companion to an existing

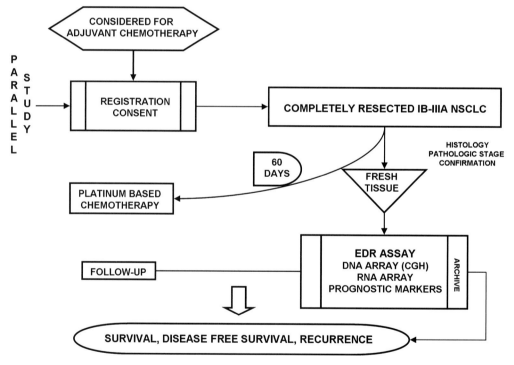

Fig. 7. A phase II validation registry trial is proposed for any patient with NSCLC where adjuvant chemotherapy is recommended, and can include inoperable stage IIIB and stage IV patients where an objective response to chemotherapy is measurable. If a parallel study exists for any NSCLC patient, they may be eligible for enrollment. As a stand-alone surgical trial, completely resected patients have viable tumor evaluated with the EDR assay. Platinum-based adjuvant chemotherapy is administered within 60 days and patients are followed for recurrence and survival end points. From archived histologically confirmed representative NSCLC tumor specimens, competitive genomic hybridization DNA arrays, RNA arrays, and prognostic immunohistochemical markers can be performed (see text). Comparisons are made between clinical end points and the in vitro assays.

adjuvant chemotherapy trial, or as a stand-alone study. Although intended for completely resected disease, unresectable advanced-stage NSCLC patients can be enrolled if their response to therapy is measurable and fresh tissue is available (Fig. 7).

A randomized prospective phase 3 trial of assay directed versus standard adjuvant chemotherapy may include patients with completely resected NSCLC, although, like a validation trial, patients with unresectable but measurable disease could be enrolled. Empiric therapy consists of a platinum doublet, and assay-directed therapy is based on the best doublet LDR combination to include a platin if the tumor is LDR to platinum. A platinum-resistant subset receives the best non-platinum based doublet or single-agent therapy.

Fresh tumor is archived for correlative studies. End points of recurrence, survival, and disease-free survival are compared between treatment arms (Fig. 8).

Summary

The frequency of in vitro chemotherapy resistance in NSCLC is extraordinary; however, its clinical relevance remains unproved. Future studies on the use of the EDR assay and its integration into clinical trials is justified. To achieve the goal "to do no harm," the EDR has a role in eliminating some ineffective agents to avoid unnecessary toxicity, and when possible, in directing

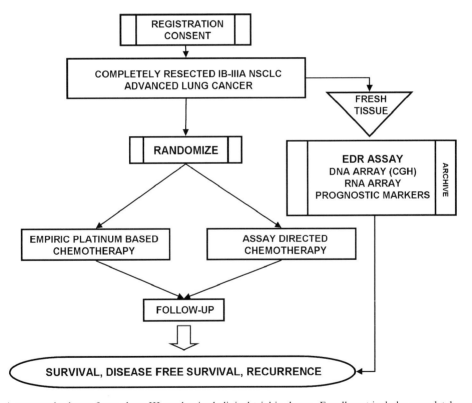

Fig. 8. A proposed schema for a phase III randomized clinical trial is shown. Enrollment includes completely resected patients with NSCLC recommended to receive adjuvant chemotherapy and can include inoperable stage IIIB and stage IV patients where objective response to chemotherapy is measurable, and resection is not indicated. All patients must have viable tissue available for the EDR assay. Archived tissue may be used for competitive genomic hybridization DNA arrays, RNA arrays, and prognostic immunohistochemical markers (see text). Patients are randomized to either a platinum-based doublet chemotherapy regimen, or chemotherapy regimen based on the results of the EDR assay. Observed outcomes of survival, overall survival, and recurrence are compared between treatment arms. The results from the EDR assay are blinded. As an intention-to-treat study, results of the EDR assay are unblinded to the treating physician in the event of recurrence. Comparisons are made between clinical response to chemotherapy and the in vitro assays for both treatment arms.

therapy. Empiric adjuvant chemotherapy for resected NSCLC may soon become passé as reproducible and generally available molecular
testing becomes more common. Profiles from
DNA and RNA expression analysis not only
help define patients at risk for early recurrence
and unresponsiveness to commonly used cytotoxic
drugs, but also assist in the development of new
assays that are less expensive, reliable, and can be
used more commonly than arrays.

References

[1] American Cancer Society. Cancer facts and figures
    2006. Atlanta: American Cancer Society; 2006.
    p. 13–5.
[2] Mountain CF. Revisions in the international system
    for staging lung cancer. Chest 1997;111:1710–7.
[3] The International Adjuvant Lung Cancer Trial
    Collaborative Group. Cisplatin-based adjuvant che-
    motherapy in patients with completely resected
    non–small-cell lung cancer. N Engl J Med 2004;
    350:351–60.
[4] Strauss GM, Herndon J, Maddaus MA, et al. Ran-
    domized clinical one page of adjuvant chemotherapy
    with paclitaxel and carboplatin following resection
    in stage IB non-small cell lung cancer (NSCLC):
    report of cancer and leukemia Group B (CALGB)
    protocol 9633. J Clin Oncol 2004;22:7019 [ASCO
    Annual Meeting Proceedings, New Orleans, Louisi-
    ana, USA].
[5] Winton TL, Livingston R, Johnson D, et al. A pro-
    spective randomised trial of adjuvant vinorelbine
    (VIN) and cisplatin (CIS) in completely resected
    stage 1B and II non small cell lung cancer (NSCLC)
    Intergroup JBR.10. N Engl J Med 2005;352:
    2289–97.
[6] Douillard J, Rosell R, Delena M, et al. ANITA:
    phase III adjuvant vinorelbine (N) and cisplatin
    (P) versus observation (OBS) in completely resected
    (stage I-III) non-small-cell lung cancer (NSCLC)
    patients (pts): final results after 70-month median
    follow-up on behalf of the Adjuvant Navelbine In-
    ternational Trialist Association. J Clin Oncol 2005;
    23:7013 [ASCO Annual Meeting Proceedings,
    Orlando, Florida, USA].
[7] Strauss G, Herndon J, Maddaus M, et al. Adjuvant
    chemotherapy in stage IB non-small cell lung cancer
    (NSCLC): update of cancer and leukemia group B
    (CALGB) protocol 9633. J Clin Oncol 2006;
    24(18S):7007 [ASCO Annual Meeting Proceedings
    Part I].
[8] Schrag D, Garewal H, Burstein H, et al. American
    Society of Clinical Oncology technology assessment:
    chemotherapy sensitivity and resistance assays.
    J Clin Oncol 2004;22:3631–8.

[9] Samson D, Seidenfeld J, Ziegler K, et al. Chemother-
    apy sensitivity and resistance assays: a systematic
    review. J Clin Oncol 2004;22:3618–30.
[10] Fruehauf J, Alberts D. In vitro drug resistance ver-
    sus chemosensitivity: two sides of different coins.
    J Clin Oncol 2005;23:3641–3.
[11] Nagourney R. Chemotherapy sensitivity and resis-
    tance assays: a systemic review? J Clin Oncol 2005;
    23:3640–1.
[12] Medicare coverage: MCAC Laboratory and Diagnos-
    tic Services Panel Human Tumor Assay Systems. Min-
    utes of November 15–16, 1999, Meeting. Available at:
    http://www.cms.hhs.gov/mcd/viewmcac.asp?where=
    basket&mid=14&basket=mcac:14:Human+Tumor+
    Assay+Systems+%28Laboratory+and+Diagnostic+
    Services+Panel%29:11/15/1999. Accessed April 23,
    2007.
[13] Fruehauf JP, Bosanquet AG. In vitro determination
    of drug response: a discussion of clinical applica-
    tions. Principles and Practice of Oncology: Updates
    1993;7(12):1–16.
[14] Kern D, Weisenthal L. Highly specific prediction of
    antineoplastic drug resistance with an in vitro assay
    using suprapharmacologic drug exposures. J Natl
    Cancer Inst 1990;82:582–8.
[15] d'Amato T, Landreneau R, McKenna R, et al. Prev-
    alence of in vitro extreme chemotherapy resistance in
    resected non-small cell lung cancer. Ann Thorac
    Surg 2006;81:440–6.
[16] d'Amato TA, Landreneau RJ, Ricketts W, et al.
    Chemotherapy resistance and oncogene expression
    in non-small cell lung cancer. J Thorac Cardiovasc
    Surg 2007;133:352–63.
[17] Mehta R, Bomstein R, Yu IR, et al. Breast cancer
    survival and in vitro tumor response in the extreme
    drug resistance assay. Breast Cancer Res Treat
    2001;66:225–37.
[18] Holloway R, Mehta R, Finkler N, et al. Association
    between in vitro platinum resistance in the EDR as-
    say and clinical outcomes for ovarian cancer pa-
    tients. Gynecol Oncol 2002;87:8–16.
[19] Loizzi V, Chan J, Osann K, et al. Survival outcomes
    in patients with recurrent ovarian cancer who were
    treated with chemoresistance assay-guided chemo-
    therapy. Am J Obstet Gynecol 2003;189:1301–7.
[20] Parker RJ, Fruehauf JP, Mehta R, et al. A pro-
    spective blinded study of predictive value of ex-
    treme drug resistance assay in patients receiving
    CPT-11 for recurrent glioma. J Neurooncol 2004;
    66:365–75.
[21] Schiller J, Harrington D, Belani C, et al. Comparison
    of four chemotherapy regimens for advanced non-
    small-cell lung cancer. N Engl J Med 2002;346:92–8.
[22] Rosell R, Cobo M, Isla D, et al. ERCC1 mRNA-
    based randomized phase III trial of docetaxel (doc)
    doublets with cisplatin (cis) or gemcitabine (gem)
    in stage IV non-small-cell lung cancer (NSCLC) pa-
    tients (p). J Clin Oncol 2005;23:7002 [ASCO Annual
    Meeting Proceedings, Orlando, Florida, USA].

[23] Olaussen KA, Dunant A, Fouret P, et al. DNA repair by ERCC1 in non-small cell lung cancer and cisplatin-based adjuvant chemotherapy. N Engl J Med 2006;355:983–91.

[24] Nevins J, Petersen R, Mukherjee S, et al. A genomic strategy to refine prognosis in early stage non-small cell lung carcinoma (NSCLC). J Clin Oncol 2006; 24(18S):7026 [ASCO Annual Meeting Proceedings Part I].

[25] Potti A, Mukherjee S, Petersen R, et al. A genomic strategy to refine prognosis in early-stage non-small cell lung cancer. N Engl J Med 2006;355: 570–80.

[26] d'Amato TA, Fernando HC, Chan BY, et al. Differential gene expression associated with early tumor recurrence and long disease free survival in early stage lung cancer. Presented at the Society of Surgical Oncology 60th Annual Meeting. Washington, DC, March 15–18, 2007.

[27] Sun Z, Yang P. Gene expression profiling on lung cancer outcome prediction: present clinical value and future premise. Cancer Epidemiol Biomarkers Prev 2006;15:2063–8.

[28] Smith DL, Shahbahrami B, Covic S, et al. Identification of amplifications and deletions in taxol resistant ovarian tumors by competitive genomic hybridization screening. Presented at the 4th International Meeting on Cancer Molecular Markers. Stone Mountain, GA, September 8–10, 2006.

[29] Wieand H. Chemotherapy sensitivity and response assays: are the ASCO guidelines for clinical trial design too restrictive? J Clin Oncol 2005;23:3643–4.

ELSEVIER
SAUNDERS

Thorac Surg Clin 17 (2007) 301–307

THORACIC
SURGERY
CLINICS

Index

Note: Page numbers of article titles are in **boldface** type.

1547-4127/07/$ - see front matter © 2007 Elsevier Inc. All rights reserved.
doi:10.1016/S1547-4127(07)00055-2

thoracic.theclinics.com

Moving?

Make sure your subscription moves with you!

To notify us of your new address, find your **Clinics Account Number** (located on your mailing label above your name), and contact customer service at:

E-mail: elspcs@elsevier.com

800-654-2452 (subscribers in the U.S. & Canada)
407-345-4000 (subscribers outside of the U.S. & Canada)

Fax number: 407-363-9661

Elsevier Periodicals Customer Service
6277 Sea Harbor Drive
Orlando, FL 32887-4800

*To ensure uninterrupted delivery of your subscription, please notify us at least 4 weeks in advance of move.